D0017585

Also by Tina Payne Bryson, Ph.D.
(with Daniel J. Siegel, M.D.)

The Whole-Brain Child
No-Drama Discipline
The Yes Brain
The Power of Showing Up

The Bottom Line for Baby

The Bottom Line for Baby

From Sleep Training to Screens, Thumb Sucking to Tummy Time— What the Science Says

TINA PAYNE BRYSON, PH.D.

BALLANTINE BOOKS
NEW YORK

No book can replace the diagnostic expertise and medical advice of a trusted physician. Please be certain to consult with your doctor before making any decisions that affect you or your family's health, particularly if you suffer from any medical condition or have any symptom that may require treatment.

A Ballantine Books Trade Paperback Original

Published in the United States by Ballantine Books, an imprint of Random House, a division of Penguin Random House LLC, New York.

LIBRARY OF CONGRESS CATALOGING-IN-PUBLICATION DATA
Names: Bryson, Tina Payne, author.
Title: The bottom line for baby / Tina Payne Bryson, Ph.D.
Description: New York: Ballantine Books, [2020] | Includes bibliographical references and index.
Identifiers: LCCN 2019053246 (print) | LCCN 2019053247 (ebook) | ISBN 9780593129968 (trade paperback; alk. paper) | ISBN 9780593129975 (ebook)
Subjects: LCSH: Infants—Care. | Infants—Development. | Parent and infant. | Infant psychology.
Classification: LCC RJ61 .B8736 2020 (print) | LCC RJ61 (ebook) | DDC 618.92/02—dc23
LC record available at https://lccn.loc.gov/2019053246
LC ebook record available at https://lccn.loc.gov/2019053247

Printed in the United States of America on acid-free paper

randomhousebooks.com

9 8 7 6 5 4 3 2 1

Book design by Diane Hobbing

For Liz:
Who always has my back, who makes me crazy laugh, who is the real treasure of every treasure hunt, and who always knows the bottom line. What would I do without you?
#NSLP

There is no other species on Earth that does science. It is, so far, entirely a human invention, evolved by natural selection in the cerebral cortex for one simple reason: it works. It's not perfect. It can be misused. It's only a tool. But it's by far the best tool we have, self-correcting, ongoing, applicable to everything.

—CARL SAGAN, *Cosmos*

Contents

Introduction

Two images come to mind when I think about the origin of this book.

The first is of a middle-aged neonatal nurse in her hospital green, checking my blood pressure mere hours after my first child was born. I'd been pestering this woman with a multitude of new-mother questions and worries—Why isn't he latching on? Is it OK to put him next to me while he's sleeping? When we get home, can our dog sleep near the crib? Then finally, in response to a question about pacifier use and nipple confusion, she stopped me by holding up her palm. Without even looking up from the pressure gauge, she told me flatly, in her West Texas accent, "Honey, look. Whatever you decide about all that stuff, he'll live."

She clearly meant well and wanted to reassure me, but I was taken aback. I didn't respond, but I remember thinking, *That's not really my goal here! Mere survival? I'm aiming higher than that.*

I didn't know exactly what it was I wanted for my new baby, but I knew it had to do with helping him be happy and healthy, both mentally and physically. I wanted him to love life and enjoy meaningful relationships, to contribute to his world. Granted, that overworked nurse didn't really mean that a parent's job was simply to help their child reach adulthood without suffering major injuries. But her comment set me exploring along a road that led to the writing of this book.

The other image I think of is from a few months later. In this one I'm sitting on the floor beside my husband in the parenting section of a bookstore in San Antonio. I don't remember what had stumped us at this particular moment, but I know that in our sleep-deprived state, we were paging through book after book as we tried to figure out how we wanted to do things for our newborn, sleeping in the stroller next to us. We felt completely overwhelmed, not only because of the sheer amount of information we encountered but also because so much of it was contradictory.

It was the same with the advice I received from everyone in my life. Our family, our friends (some with kids and some without), a random woman at a restaurant, the produce guy at the grocery store—it seemed like everyone I met had advice about what I should do with my son. Though it was obviously well intended, their input was sometimes outdated, often unhelpful, and, again, consistently contradictory. One person said I should sleep with my baby. Another warned that I shouldn't even talk to him at night, much less hold him. One person urged me to get him on a schedule right away. Another stressed that I should simply respond to his needs and requests. The information storm left me feeling completely untethered.

Now, twenty years later, I'm the mother of three boys, I'm a trained mental health and child development professional, and I've built a career studying, researching, writing, and talking with other parents about the joys and struggles of raising kids. I've read article after article in scientific journals from many different fields of study, as well as from popular parenting magazines and online sources. I've read countless parenting and child development books. And over the last few years I've written several parenting books with my good friend, mentor, and colleague Dan Siegel. For me it's been a quest to find out what's most important when raising children—so that we can help them do a lot more than just survive.

Based on what I've learned from my own reading and research, and from talking to parents about what works best for them, it's clear that one of the primary challenges of raising a child is gathering the best possible information from trusted sources, considering your child's individual uniqueness, and then listening to your instincts, values, and principles. But that's not easy when you're faced with the astounding volume of parenting information online, fed to you via social media and often written in a provocative, clickbait kind of way. How are you supposed to know which information is accurate and trustworthy?

What I want to do here is help you wade through the cacophony of voices clamoring to tell you what to do with your baby. I'll help you discover the most up-to-date information about the issues and questions you're facing so that you can make the best decisions about your child. In the coming pages we'll tackle together the most common, critical, controversial, and confusing questions that new parents wrestle with—related to breastfeeding, sleep scheduling, vaccinations, discipline, and whatever else you're wondering and worrying about. My goal is to provide you with clear, accessible information based on the latest science, and for each individual topic I aim to demystify the issue so that you can concentrate on what matters most and more easily make your best decisions for your family.

Notice that I keep talking about which decisions *you,* the mom or dad (or grandparent or other primary caregiver), make. Families come in all shapes and sizes, and there's rarely a one-size-fits-all set of data that answers all questions for all families. My goal is therefore to provide you with the information that lets you make your own best decision. *Of course* it's helpful to listen to experts and consider science when making decisions about your child. That's the fundamental principle this whole book is based on. Knowledge is power, and most of us step into parenting not knowing much about all the details and decisions and options and science available to us. That's why we listen to others. And yes, it's important that you question your own preconceived opinions and biases when faced with new information.

But ultimately, this is *your* baby and *your* family that you're deciding about. I've worked hard to maintain an awareness of and sensitivity to the fact that different traditions and cultures will approach various child-rearing ideas differently; and still, I'm approaching the subjects in this book from my own perspective, with my own assumptions. You'll have to do the same with the questions you face. Every child and parent and family constellation is unique, and there's no "right" way to do family. Whatever your culture and family makeup, it's important to have credible information. Then you can consider your traditions and values, paying attention to your parental instincts and your child's unique and ever-changing individual needs. When all of that comes together, you can make the decisions that make the most sense for your child, yourself, and your family.

The Organization of This Book

THIS BOOK'S FOCUS is on questions about *babies,* which I'm defining as children twelve months or younger. At times I'll discuss older children as well, but primarily I'll be highlighting issues as they pertain to your infant's first year.

And let me be clear: this is not a how-to guide. The point is not to give instructions for dealing with various issues that come up—treating a fever, choosing a crib, recognizing diaper rash, maintaining parental self-care, and so on. There are lots of good books out there that do just that, many of which I recommend all the time. The point here isn't to present an exhaustive collection of *every question* new parents will ask. Instead, it's an attempt to address virtually all the main *dilemmas* new parents will face, where they receive competing advice from the people around them.

I've organized the material alphabetically, so you can easily look up subjects you're wondering about. Or you might prefer to read through from beginning to end. Either way, you'll see quickly that each entry in this book—covering topics from alcohol and antibiotics to vaping and walkers—is organized around three main sections: "Competing Opinions," "What the Science Says," and "The Bottom Line." The first section quickly and objectively summarizes different perspectives or schools of thought related to the present subject. Your mother-in-law, for example, might be a huge fan of swaddling a baby and wants to show you how. But maybe your brother says he's read a recent article suggesting that swaddling leads to sudden infant death syndrome (SIDS). The advice from each person generally makes sense—to them, at least, and maybe to you as well. This is the type of challenge new parents so often find themselves faced with.

It's not that there are necessarily only two perspectives on each topic, by the way, or that I want to oversimplify complicated parenting dilemmas into cable-TV-style "pro/con" debates. But I've found through my years of working with parents that it's often helpful to set the parameters of the discussion in this way, then dig into the gray areas from there. In doing so here, I've worked to avoid setting up any one perspective as an oversimplified "straw man" position; my goal is to present each opinion as persuasively as possible, creating a situation that mimics the actual dilemmas you face.

When more than two perspectives need to be considered, or the issue is just too complex to be broken down into binary positions, I've divided it into multiple entries. With childcare, for instance, you'll see one entry on the effects of working outside the home, and a different one on choosing between center-based daycare and nannies. Likewise, on the subject of scheduling and babies, you'll find entries on sleep training, baby-led weaning, extended breastfeeding, and on-demand feeding. The goal is to simplify things for you, but to do so without oversimplifying the actual data and information.

After the "Competing Opinions" section, each entry then offers "What the Science Says." Here I offer a focused, simplified summary of the conclusions the scientific community has drawn regarding that particular issue. Some entries are longer than others, depending on the complexity of the topic and the depth of the body of research. But throughout, I've prioritized making sure that the information you encounter is not only accurate but concise as well. If you're the parent of a young child, you are by definition already stretched thin, so I've worked to make it easy on you to quickly get an overview of the research literature on each topic. If you're interested in reading the specifics of the science, or if you'd like to take a deeper dive, the bibliography is a great place to start.

Finally, after presenting the research summary, each entry will offer "The Bottom Line," where I boil down the prior information and offer an overall "Here's what it all comes down to" message. The bottom line of a particular entry may be that the science is clear about which approach is best for kids. Or it may be that the science hasn't yet clearly or conclusively addressed that issue, in which case families should simply follow common sense along with their instincts and cultural values. Other times the bottom line will be that the science is contradictory or weak and doesn't provide helpful guidance at all. My constant invitation will be for you to become informed, then apply the science in a way that's consistent with what you believe and what you want for your child, yourself, and your family.

That's what I've tried to do with my own family. And as you'll see, in some entries I've added a personal note, where I weigh in about my personal feelings, experiences, and even biases when it comes to a given topic.

Speaking of biases, I want to state from the outset that my starting position when it comes to anything regarding child rearing is that it essentially comes down to relationship. While we always have to be careful about saying there's "one answer" to anything having to do with a subject as complex as parenting, I'm a firm believer that what a child needs more than anything is the love and attention of a committed caregiver. That's what best develops their brains and the essence of who they become. Aside from safety, sleep, and nutrition, nothing's more important than having a caregiver who is fully present and attentive to the child's needs, attuning and responding to what's being communicated. Gadgets and enrichment classes may make things more convenient and fun, but what's most important for children is having adults in their lives who tune in to their needs and respond accordingly.

A Few Words About the Science

WE LIVE IN an exciting time, when science is helping inform us and answer many of our most important questions. That certainly applies to parenting. A foundational assumption of this book is that we should be guided by the best available information regarding the various dilemmas we face as we raise our kids.

That said, it's important to keep in mind that contemporary scientific knowledge is very much a work in progress. There's a seemingly infinite amount of information about the world that science hasn't figured out yet. Likewise, conclusions drawn by research might be working from incomplete evidence or based on limited and/or flawed studies. Or the researchers might be biased or compromised in some way, either because of financial considerations or because of self-interest. There's even good science following best practices that may still be proven wrong or wanting by better measures in the future.

What's more, the research we're typically discussing when it comes to parenting focuses on human beings, who are complex and can't always be put into neat little categories. Most studies typically base their analyses, and therefore their conclusions and interpretations, on discrete categories. Even simple answers to straightforward questions don't always yield a complete picture. For instance, a researcher might ask a parent, "Do you let your child watch TV?" The available answers might be "Yes" or "No," or "Choose a number between 1 and 5, with 1 being 'never' and 5 being 'all the time.' " While those responses can capture a good amount of information, there's not a box that lets you answer, "Well, it depends on whether my child already went on a playdate that day and needs a break, or whether she was at her cousin's house, where I know she already had screen time." That kind of complexity is difficult to get at with interview questions.

Does that mean we can't trust science? Of course not. It would be ridiculous to deny the most complete information we currently have, produced by decades of replicated research, and instead make decisions based on our predetermined opinions and biases. Rather, we want to rely on the science, but approach it humbly. We want to make decisions by informing ourselves with the best studies out there—the ones written by trusted experts, reviewed by their peers, published in respected journals, and endorsed by leading health organizations. At times the available research can lead us to confident conclusions; in other situations it will offer mere guidance, leaving us to consider incomplete or even conflicting evidence. Then we use our best judgment, considering our values and the unique needs and temperaments of our family.

You might make a call that goes against research because it fits your current situation, your family's needs, or your child's personality. Let's say you read the entry here about the many benefits children receive when there's a pet in the home. But if one of your older kids is allergic to dogs, you might forgo this particular advantage for your baby. Or if your spouse is in the military and stationed far away, you might loosen the screen time reins so that your infant gets to interact with his parent on a regular basis. The point is that while we allow science to guide us, we don't want to become overly rigid in our devotion to it.

It's also important that we evaluate science with discretion. A study's methodology should be sound, with a meaningful number of appropriate subjects, clear parameters and definitions, and a duration long enough to measure the pattern the researchers discover. Then in interpreting results, we want to recognize the difference between correlation and causation. A child who lives in a big house might read at a higher level than one in a smaller house, but that doesn't mean that the size of the house is *causing* the improved reading skills. I've taken factors such as these into account as I considered, sifted through, and summarized the research, but for the most part I won't be getting too far into the methodological weeds in my discussion of the research.

When they're available, I've relied heavily on recent meta-analyses because they typically remove poor-quality studies, pulling together investigations with strong methodology, consistent and theory-driven definitions, and valid measures. Then they summarize or analyze the convergence of the findings of the valid, relevant data in order to determine—with much more credibility—the conclusions of the methodologically sound studies, taken together. I've also prioritized the opinions of respected professional organizations such as the American Academy of Pediatrics (AAP), the Centers for Disease Control and Prevention (CDC), and the World Health Organization (WHO). These organizations and others rely on teams of smart, educated, experienced professionals who comb through the latest research in order to offer their policy statements. While you or I might not agree with all of their conclusions and recommendations, they are important sources of the latest summary of the science.

And finally, I've relied on colleagues around the world who have graciously given their time to weigh in on the science I've presented here. Since it's impossible for me to be an expert on every topic in the book, I'm grateful to the many researchers, pediatricians, child development experts, and other professionals whose guidance I leaned on and who helped me hone and clarify the information I'm sharing with you so it's as accurate and well-defined as possible. (See the acknowledgments for more details.)

To be clear, I'm not providing here a comprehensive listing of every research study ever performed on a given subject. I'm a trained researcher who geeks out on research and information, and as I wrote this book I sometimes found it difficult to summarize succinctly the ever-evolving and complex available material. I wanted to tell you *everything*, including each minor detail or possibly confounding piece of evidence. But then I'd remind myself, "That's not what this book is," and I'd return to my focus of performing a comprehensive literature review and summarizing relevant, quality findings in a short-form way that I hope will be both compelling and helpful, as well as easy for the average parent to digest.

I've worked hard to maintain an awareness of and sensitivity to the fact that our different traditions and cultures, socioeconomic histories, and even our geographies influence our various child-rearing ideas and practices. Since this book is translated into other languages and sold in countries around the world, I want to take a moment to note that I'm aware that I am both influenced and limited by growing up in my own culture, with a certain amount of privilege, and by living in and raising children only in the United States.

I want to acknowledge as well that this book doesn't present information you couldn't obtain on your own. I've simply done the legwork for you. Some of this data you could find for yourself merely by googling and wading through various sources to determine which ones are trustworthy. For some of the information, you'd need access to an academic library and its databases. But ultimately, I'm not giving you any sort of "behind the curtain" knowledge that only "parenting experts" know about. I'm also not a physician, and I'm not giving medical advice. As always, any important health-related decisions should be discussed with your pediatrician. I'm simply assembling the information and offering it in a way that I hope will make your life easier and give you more time to be with your little one (or to take a quick nap or get a snack or go to the bathroom, for goodness' sake!).

A Final Promise

I'VE HELD YOU in mind as I've written this book, working hard to make sure that what follows won't beat you down with lists of more stuff you should be doing, or make you feel guilty about the way you parent. The last thing any of us needs is to feel more pressure or judgment about the way we're raising our kids. Too many books leave us walking away feeling "I need to be more . . ." or "I need to do more . . ." None of us will ever be a perfect parent. Even when it comes to the topics I've covered here, you're not going to get them all "right" or even do what's "best" in every scenario. That's impossible.

Some of the suggestions in this book are actually mutually exclusive! You'll learn, for instance, that it's "best" for parents to be well rested, since it reduces their risk for depression. But it's also beneficial to breastfeed your infant, who at least as a newborn, needs to eat every couple of hours, all through the night. All the choices we make have intended and unintended consequences. If you choose to nurse throughout the night on a regular basis, you're going to miss out on a lot of crucial sleep and may be more frustrated and less patient with your kids during the day. So your baby gets the benefit of breastfeeding, but you may be a little grumpier. Alternatively, you're more rested and patient, but not nursing at night. The point is simply that the decisions we make while parenting are multidimensional and interconnected like a web, and we can't achieve everything we want. You might be a firm believer that the best caretaker for an infant is the baby's parent, but you also believe in socializing her so that she's comfortable being held by other people, and that can't happen if you spend every second holding her yourself and never allow others to take care of her.

Good parenting typically requires flexibility and compromise as we decide which parts of which priorities get emphasized in our unique families and which parts get left by the wayside. We're constantly trying to strike a good balance between what we know are nonnegotiables (like car seats, pool safety, and emotional responsiveness) and what we'd like to do but simply can't. In this book you'll find all kinds of information about screen time, potty training, bug spray, probiotics, thumb sucking, and on and on. Can you cover it all and make sure everything is "perfect" in your baby's childhood? Of course not. Will you make mistakes along the way? Of course you will. We all do, even when we have good instincts and information. The ultimate goal is to cover enough of the important stuff while realizing that you can't be perfect and you can't do everything. And along the way, you nurture your baby as much as you possibly can, both physically and emotionally. If you do that, she'll do much more than just live.

In the end, quality parenting is not about raising superkids, and it's not about creating a valedictorian, a beauty pageant winner, or a major-league shortstop. We can do tremendous harm when we put undue pressure on ourselves and our kids to be the best at everything. And I definitely won't be telling you, except when the science is clear and robust, that there's "one true way" to handle a situation. The fact is that in most cases, there are lots of ways to be good parents, and even when we don't *do* what's "best," we can still be the best parents we can be. I have friends who make decisions that are very different from what my husband and I do when it comes to child rearing. Some of those differences are minor, and some are pretty significant. And guess what? We have great (but not perfect) kids, and they have great (but not perfect) kids, too! Parents tend to feel strongly on bigger issues, and there can be a lot of judgment hurled toward those who stray from what we think best. But over time I've seen again and again that even when families approach child rearing from different perspectives, they can all raise kids who are happy and healthy, ready to live meaningful lives.

I hope this book can also help you get all the various caregivers in your child's life on the same page. If a babysitter or grandparent insists, for example, that your baby shouldn't play in the sandbox at the neighborhood park because of the dirt and germs, you can turn to the entry on germs and point to the science showing that exposure to dirt helps build the immune system. (This approach to sharing the information might be more effective and provoke less conflict than just telling your mother-in-law or your intrusive neighbor to pipe down.) Or if you have friends who advise avoiding baby talk, turn to the entry on "parentese" and find out what the research says. Used as a tool for updating outdated information or beliefs and correcting false assumptions, this book can support you with the latest science and reduce battles over parenting decisions.

Ultimately, knowledge is power. Inform yourself. Then trust yourself. You know your child better than anyone. Yes, of course, you have to watch out for your own personal biases; my assumption here is that you're truly, sincerely listening to and considering what the science and experts tell you. But once you've done that, your instincts will often tell you how to respond to your baby's needs, and those instincts are there for a reason. What your child requires most is not a perfect parent (as if there were such a being), but a loving, knowledgeable, and flexible caregiver who does their best to recognize and respond to his needs quickly and consistently based on the best available information. That's the bottom line.

The Bottom Line for Baby

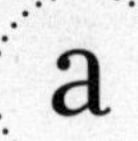

Alcohol and Breastfeeding

Is it OK to drink alcohol while nursing?

Competing Opinions

Perspective #1: Just as you wouldn't consume alcohol while pregnant, you don't want your newborn to ingest it through breast milk.

Perspective #2: Responsible drinking won't hurt the baby. Life is already restrictive enough for nursing mothers. There's no good reason to take away something else.

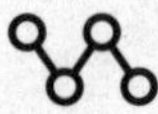

What the Science Says

SINCE THE SCIENTIFIC literature regarding this question is still evolving, it's difficult to draw a clear line in the sand. If you want to eliminate all risk, the safest approach is not to drink at all when you're nursing. But there is scant scientific evidence that drinking alcohol poses a risk to a breastfeeding baby. Many health organizations and regulatory authorities still take what one article calls a "better safe than sorry" approach and recommend drinking only in moderation. According to the CDC, moderate alcohol consumption—defined as one standard drink per day—is not known to be harmful to a newborn, especially if the mother waits a couple of hours after drinking it before nursing. The AAP agrees and states that "ingestion of alcoholic beverages should be minimized and limited to an occasional intake," specifying that it should be no more than "approximately 2 oz liquor, 8 oz wine, or 2 beers."

Exposure to more than this moderate amount has the potential to negatively affect not only growing babies' development and growth but also their sleep patterns. And, contrary to certain previous beliefs that alcohol increases milk production, studies show that it can actually limit the let-down reflex (although this is compensated for in the following hours by the baby consuming more). It's worth noting, too, that expressing milk and then discarding it may not prevent the baby from ingesting any alcohol. The alcohol level in breast milk is based on the amount of alcohol in the mother's bloodstream. The idea that the baby's exposure is eliminated if you use the "pump and dump" method is outdated, and that's no longer considered the safest way to prevent alcohol from being in your breast milk. As long as you have alcohol in your bloodstream, it can also be in your breast milk. So if you drink more than a moderate amount and your blood alcohol content is high (say, at a wedding or other celebration), it's safest to feed your baby stored milk or formula in the meantime before breastfeeding again hours later.

Finally, and not insignificantly, too much alcohol can obviously impair a mother's ability to be present to her baby's needs and make good decisions as she takes care of her infant.

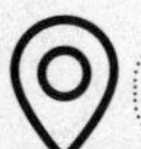

The Bottom Line

IT MAY SURPRISE you, but ultimately there's no evidence that drinking in moderation is going to harm your breastfed child, especially if you take necessary precautions. According to the AAP and the CDC, you can have a drink, wait a couple of hours, and then nurse. If you follow that recommendation, you don't have to worry that your baby will ingest the alcohol through your breast milk. If you want to be extra cautious, you can pump milk beforehand and use the stored milk when it's time to nurse. Some mothers may feel more comfortable not taking any risk and choose to forgo all alcoholic drinks until they stop nursing. Others, though, will want to have a glass of wine on the (rare?) night out, or a beer at the end of a (much less rare) exhausting day.

a

Antibiotics

Antibiotics are the most common drugs used for children in Western countries. They offer clear benefits, but science has demonstrated definite downsides as well. Are they safe for babies?

Competing Opinions

Perspective #1: Research has linked antibiotics to all kinds of health problems, and they're particularly dangerous for kids. Antibiotics kill bacteria but are useless in treating viruses, and it's often difficult to distinguish between bacterial and viral infections in infants, especially those under three months. So doctors will often overprescribe antibiotics "just to be safe," meaning that babies might be taking a powerful and potentially dangerous medicine for no reason at all.

Perspective #2: Yes, antibiotics come with a certain amount of risk. But without them, infections could potentially get worse and worse. As with any other medicine, parents should be judicious with the use of antibiotics and follow a doctor's lead when they are prescribed. But they are absolutely necessary in many situations, and the benefits outweigh the dangers.

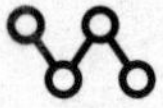

What the Science Says

ANTIBIOTICS ARE EXTREMELY effective at killing bacteria and can effectively treat common childhood bacterial infections such as strep throat, urinary tract infections, and recurring or severe ear infections. But like any medication, they can present problems as well. For example, 10 percent of children who take antibiotics will experience side effects including rashes, allergic reactions, nausea, diarrhea, and stomach pain. Antibiotics have also been linked to childhood obesity, metabolic and immunological diseases, asthma, and bowel disorders, and they've been associated with a long-lasting shift in microbiota composition and metabolism that affects the childhood microbiome and its ability to prevent disease.

These are particularly concerning realities considering how often antibiotics are overprescribed; the CDC estimates that 30 percent of antibiotic prescriptions are "inappropriate" and unnecessary. The most common example is when they are used in an attempt to treat not bacteria but a virus, against which they are unlikely to have any effect. Antibiotics wouldn't alleviate symptoms from a sore throat caused by a common cold virus, for example. So when children are unnecessarily treated with antibiotics, they are at risk of suffering the abovementioned negative outcomes without reason.

In addition, when doctors overprescribe antibiotics, the risk increases that diseases will become resistant to the drugs through repeated exposure. The WHO and others have warned about the development of antibiotic resistance and labeled it a global health concern, noting that it can significantly compromise the ability to treat infections.

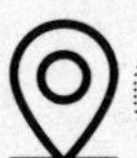

The Bottom Line

ANTIBIOTICS ARE A valuable tool that can fight illness and save lives. Some infections, if left untreated, will only get worse and can be dangerous. So be careful about letting the pendulum swing so far that you swear off antibiotics even when they're actually needed to help your infant get well. But be mindful that these medicines are regularly overprescribed. Overuse of antibiotics can make them less effective, and could potentially even produce harmful, long-lasting changes in your child's immune system, gut, and metabolism.

Educate yourself about when antibiotics should be given so that you can ask the right questions and have a more productive conversation with your pediatrician when your child is sick. Ask about the specific bacteria being addressed or the overall strategy being employed. It's great to have a trustworthy doctor whose approach is aligned with yours, and it's also essential that you two communicate and work together to make informed decisions you're both comfortable with.

On a Personal Note

WHEN I WAS a new mother, I did my best to educate myself about the differences between bacterial infections and viruses and to read up on symptoms my kids had. And still, most of the time, I just decided to trust my pediatrician. Not that a baby is a car, but when my mechanic tells me my exhaust manifold gasket (Is that a real thing?) needs to be replaced, there's not a whole lot I can do to evaluate his advice. Likewise, when my pediatrician says my infant has an infection and needs an antibiotic, I trust her perspective. I ask questions, but at the end of the day, I have to decide whether to go with my trusted physician's advice or follow my often fear-based, shallow, "I play a doctor on TV" opinion.

When you choose a pediatrician, pick someone you feel good about trusting. There will be times when you're so tired from caring for a sick infant that you'll need to rely on your doctor to think clearly and make calls that you can follow.

Baby-Led Weaning When Introducing Solids

Baby-led weaning (BLW) is quickly growing in popularity these days. The name might make you think it's about allowing your baby to determine when you stop breastfeeding, but actually, it refers to an approach to starting solid foods once the baby is around six months. Breast milk or formula remains the primary source of nutrition, but when it's time to introduce solid foods, you jump past the puree stage and go straight to finger foods. (The approach began in the United Kingdom, where "weaning" means adding complementary foods, rather than giving up nursing, which is the primary definition in the United States.)

The basic idea is that once your baby is old enough to spoon-feed herself and can safely munch soft bites of healthy foods, you let her take a more active role in her eating. That means you get to bypass much of the spoon-feeding phase, and instead of relying on diluted cereal and pureed food (whether jarred or homemade), you set out finger foods—often cut-up pieces of what everyone else at the family table is having—and allow your child to take the lead in her own feeding process.

Are there risks involved, in terms of your infant's health, nutrition, and overall development? Is BLW worth doing, or is there reason to be wary of this recent trend?

Competing Opinions

Perspective #1: BLW comes with many benefits, like learning to chew and developing manual dexterity and hand-eye coordination. It also has the potential to offer babies different kinds of flavors and textures beyond purees, meaning that they're learning from the get-go to be more flexible and even adventurous with what they'll eat. Exposure to many different kinds of foods can reduce allergies down the road as well. The other key advantage is that with BLW, kids learn to regulate their own food intake based on hunger, rather than having parents decide how much they eat. As a result, they'll be less prone later in life to diet-related problems such as obesity.

Perspective #2: BLW can be messy and time-consuming, but it also poses a problem because it can make it difficult to know whether your baby will get what she needs nutritionally. When you spoon-feed infants, you can know exactly what's going in and whether it's the right amount to ensure health; that means you can help them maintain a healthy weight. With BLW, though, you're often left wondering whether your child is eating her food or just playing with it. The other primary concern is that BLW comes with an increased risk of choking.

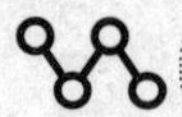

What the Science Says

WHILE STUDIES HAVE found evidence backing the claims of BLW proponents, these studies have their methodological limitations. When it comes to a comparison between spoon-fed and baby-led feeding, reliable studies find almost nothing remarkable in terms of long-term outcomes. One set of researchers did report that kids whose parents practiced BLW showed a stronger preference for fruits and vegetables at the age of two, and another found that parents of BLW children reported less food fussiness and greater enjoyment of food at twelve months. But otherwise there weren't notable differences between the groups.

Still, when considering BLW, parents and authorities express concerns regarding three dynamics: the possibility of choking, reduced iron intake, and slower growth among babies feeding themselves. Because of these apprehensions, a modified BLW process—the BLISS method (baby-led introduction to solids)—has been recommended. The BLISS method adjusts conventional BLW by enhancing the iron intake and guiding parents toward foods with a lower choking risk. Some early results point to the success of the BLISS method, but sufficient evidence has yet to be established by the scientific community. For example, one investigation found that the modified BLW approach, where parents were advised on how to minimize choking risks, did reduce that risk, so those children were no more likely to choke than infants following "more traditional feeding practices." But the authors of the study still felt the need to declare that "the large number of children in both groups offered foods that pose a choking risk is concerning."

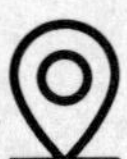

The Bottom Line

WITH LIMITED EVIDENCE currently available to recommend baby-led introduction of solid foods, it's a good idea to proceed with caution, primarily regarding choking and proper nutrition and weight gain. But these are concerns worthy of careful attention no matter what. (See the entry "Introducing Solid Foods.")

At this point, there doesn't seem to be enough evidence to positively persuade you to try BLW or dissuade you from going that route. In a few years we'll know more. But if you'd like to skip the mashed-peas phase, or at least move toward a hybrid approach where you introduce more finger foods as well, then it should be safe—and it might be fun—to allow your little one to sit in her high chair and share in the family meal from time to time. As always, make your decision after discussing it with your pediatrician, who can help assess your baby's overall development and readiness for solid foods.

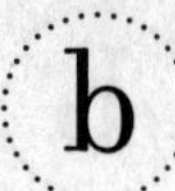

Baby Powder

Is it safe to use baby powder?

Competing Opinions

Perspective #1: Baby powder absorbs moisture and decreases friction that results from a baby's skin rubbing against a diaper. It's one of the best tools you can use to combat diaper rash. That's why it's been relied on by parents for decades.

Perspective #2: It's true that baby powder has been used for years, but we now know that it's dangerous for infants. The talc in the powder can be inhaled by a baby and significantly damage his lungs. It might even cause cancer.

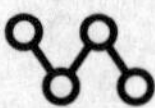

What the Science Says

ACCORDING TO THE American Academy of Pediatrics, moms and dads should avoid using baby powder of any kind. It's not necessary, and worse, it can be extremely dangerous. If an infant inhales particles of a talcum-containing powder, it can cause severe lung damage and breathing problems. And respiratory issues aren't the only risk. The American Cancer Society has issued a statement asserting an association between talc and ovarian cancer when the powder comes into contact with the genital area.

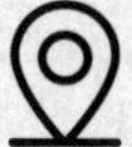

The Bottom Line

STAY AWAY FROM baby powder. I know you might associate it with the classic baby scent, but it's dangerous for your child. Talc-free powders do exist, but even a cornstarch-based powder can cause breathing problems if it's inhaled. What's more, you don't need the powder. There are safer, more effective ways to deal with diaper rash: change diapers promptly when they're wet or dirty, gently clean your baby's bottom with fragrance-free wipes or a moist cloth, dry the skin (or let it air-dry) before putting on a new diaper, and use a diaper ointment if your infant regularly gets rashes. These are best practices that can keep you from needing to use powder at all.

If you've already been using baby powder with your infant, you don't need to feel guilty or anxious. But now you know there are safer options to keep your baby fresh and rash free.

b

Babywearing

In recent decades, babywearing—the practice of "wearing" or carrying an infant in some sort of carrier, like a wrap or a sling—has become more and more popular in the United States. While the practice has been popular in other cultures around the world for centuries, some worry about its effects on a baby's physical health, as well as how it might affect the parent-child relationship.

Competing Opinions

Perspective #1: Babywearing is a great way to increase closeness with your baby. It allows you to remain attuned and cued to his needs, while letting him attune to you and your movements, all of which reduces his stress and keeps him from being as fussy. This feedback loop, where he lets you know that he's hungry, bored, or wet and you are able to respond right away, will also increase the trust in the relationship. Babywearing can be especially powerful for dads, partners, grandparents, and other caregivers who aren't getting the additional bonding experiences that can come with breastfeeding. It's also convenient, since it allows you to take care of other children or accomplish various chores while remaining connected to your infant and keeping him happier.

Perspective #2: There are plenty of ways to be close with your baby without wearing him around. If you carry him everywhere, you could inhibit his desire to learn to crawl or walk. Plus, when he does stand on his own, he might be less independent and become clingy since he's used to having you holding him all the time. You can also cause hip, knee, spine, neck, and circulation problems with improper positioning, and back pain for yourself. What's worse, wearing your baby can lead to constriction, overheating, and even suffocation.

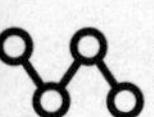

What the Science Says

NUMEROUS STUDIES HAVE demonstrated the many benefits of frequent holding and skin-to-skin contact with babies. While babywearing typically isn't done skin to skin, it could include "supplemental carrying," which means holding and carrying babies beyond the typical amount that takes place during feeding or in response to crying. Studies have observed that infants carried by a walking mother as opposed to being held by a sitting mother will cry less, be more still, and have a slower heart rate. To explain this calming effect, researchers point to the coordination of the central, motor, and cardiac systems that occurs when a mother walks while holding her child. (These studies were performed by looking at mother-infant interactions, but presumably the results would be similar with fathers.)

Studies have shown abundant benefits of babywearing, even without the direct skin-to-skin contact. Breastfeeding rates increase and infant stomachaches can occur less regularly. The spitting up, coughing, and breathing problems that come with gastroesophageal reflux were significantly mitigated when infants were monitored in an upright position (as would be the case when they are worn) rather than lying down. What's more, babywearing can promote bonding and possibly even stimulate physical growth, especially among preterm babies. The skin-to-skin contact also has the potential to reduce postpartum depression in the mother. In addition, research has found that certain types of massage therapy can promote physical growth, and while it hasn't been proven that wearing a baby offers similar benefits, some suggest that the moderate pressure of being in a sling could have some of the benefits of massage therapy, particularly when parents are also touching the baby's feet, hands, arms, head, and back while wearing the child.

Despite these benefits, it's also true that babywearing comes with certain risks, including poor alignment, circulation, and overheating for the baby, along with back pain for the caregiver. Proponents point out, though, that these hazards can be largely avoided by practicing certain rules of thumb (discussed in the next section).

One concern you don't have to worry about is that holding your baby a lot and creating this kind of consistent closeness will make him clingy or dependent. (See the entry "Discipline.") Decades of scientific research have demonstrated that responsive parental attunement leads to kids becoming *more* independent and self-sufficient, not less.

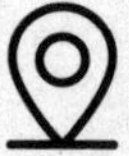

The Bottom Line

WHEN DONE CORRECTLY and safely, babywearing can be good for both you and your baby. It has the potential to reduce crying and make colic more manageable, promote close bonding and secure attachment (which can increase cognitive and social development), help your baby feel safe and calm, allow you greater freedom to work on daily tasks or parent other children while keeping your infant safe and happy, reduce postnatal depression and anxiety, and even promote and prolong breastfeeding relationships.

Even with this list of benefits, don't feel like you have to wear your baby all the time, or do it for the entirety of the first year. It can be hot, uncomfortable, and tiresome for the parent, particularly as the baby grows, so use good sense and take care of your own needs as well. At some point, when your tiny infant with cute little swinging legs becomes a huge, heavy child whose long legs are kicking hard, you might decide that babywearing is no longer for you.

It's worth remembering, too, that while there are obvious benefits to wearing babies in carriers like a wrap or a sling, infants can fall, be injured, and even die in their parent's sling. According to the U.S. Consumer Product Safety Commission, seventeen babies died between 2003 and 2016 while being worn in infant carriers. Experts have therefore de-

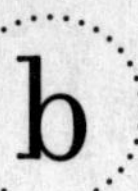

veloped an acronym, known as the TICKS rules, to help you remember the key babywearing priorities: Tight (snug) slings and carriers, In view at all times (your baby should face you), Close enough to kiss, Keep chin off chest, and Support baby's back. Be sure, too, to avoid cooking or working near a stove while wearing your baby. And as always, you should consult your pediatrician if you're unsure or need further guidance.

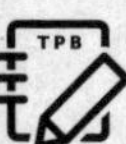

On a Personal Note

I LOVED BABYWEARING and found it useful in a practical sense, as it freed up my hands, especially when I was caring for my other children. But I also felt good knowing that my baby, especially during those first few months, felt so much more comfortable and safe next to me.

There were times, though, as my babies got bigger, that it completely exhausted me. I'm 5'4" but my husband is 6'2", so we had long and tall children. As much as my babies or I might have liked them in the BabyBjörn or the wrap, this just stopped working for my body. (I admit I love gear, so I always had several options for strapping my baby onto me.) Plus, I'm sure it looked silly to have a small mom toting a baby whose legs almost hit her knees. I started using the stroller a lot more.

Each kid is different, too. One of my boys would have let us carry or push him around well into childhood—he liked the ride! But eventually he was so tall that he was kicking my husband in places that might have prevented us from having additional children, so that chapter came to a close.

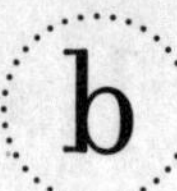

Bathing

Bathing your newborn or young infant may seem straightforward, but questions and differences of opinion often arise regarding the type and frequency of baths.

Competing Opinions

Perspective #1: Babies should have only sponge baths until the stump of the umbilical cord falls off; for a circumcised boy, sponge baths only until the site completely heals. (See "First Bath.") Using a gentle cloth for a newborn's face, hands, and bottom is more than enough to keep your baby clean. As for how often, there's really no need to bathe newborns daily, particularly if they have dry or sensitive skin. Even older babies don't generally need to be bathed more than three times a week.

Perspective #2: If your baby enjoys his bath or finds it soothing, there's no harm in daily bathing right away. And as he gets older, bath time can become part of the bedtime routine and help calm and relax him for the night.

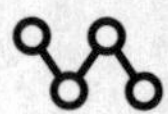

What the Science Says

THE AAP RECOMMENDS, and most evidence supports, sponge baths until the stump of the umbilical cord falls off and, for a circumcised boy, until the wound heals. Most experts agree that it's not necessary to bathe a newborn every day. Two or three times a week should be plenty, and really, throughout the first year three baths a week may be enough. More than that risks drying out the baby's skin, especially if you use harsh soaps. An infant's skin is sensitive and hasn't had time yet to develop the ability to maintain moisture, so the skin can easily become dry and irritated. This can be particularly true for African American and some biracial infants, whose skin is prone to dryness and sensitivity.

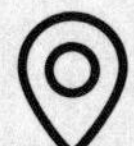

The Bottom Line

THERE'S NO NEED to make sure your baby gets a daily bath as long as you're keeping him clean and washing his diaper area when you change him. You'll have plenty of time down the road to incorporate a bath into the bedtime routine. For now, it's best to limit baths to two or three times per week most of the time. If, however, you're a parent who tolerates or even encourages messy play and exploration, or if your family includes pets or siblings who get dirty and like to snuggle with your baby, you may need to add a bath or two. Be mindful of your infant's sensitive skin, set a general rule of two to three times per week, and then use your judgment.

One other point: Most babies and toddlers enjoy bath time, as it's typically a pleasant, relaxing sensory experience. But for some babies and toddlers, baths or water experiences are really unpleasant, even painful for them. For kids who have sensory integration challenges, bath time can be full of frustration, fear, and even screaming. The water's too hot, cold, low, high, fast, slow, and on and on. If this is your experience, learn more about sensory processing at SPDstar.org.

On a Personal Note

I LOVED THE bath time part of the day with my babies and toddlers. They were (usually) happy, fun, and engaged. It was a great time to make up silly songs and connect. And what's more delicious than a slippery, sweet-smelling, freshly bathed baby? (Can you tell I still have baby fever?)

To this day, one of my favorite baby gifts for new parents, along with some books, is a foam gardening pad; meant for comfort while weeding or planting, it is the perfect support for your knees next to the bath as well. It's much more comfortable than kneeling on a towel, and because it's meant for outdoor use, it can get wet. Eventually, toddlers and preschoolers can use the pad for fun in the tub because it floats and they can put toys on it like a little water table. Easy and inexpensive!

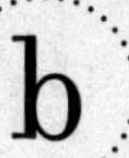

Bilingualism

Parents of children in bilingual households, and those who want to teach their infant a second language at an early age, often have questions about the advantages and disadvantages of the bilingual experience. Will it be beneficial for their child, or will it confuse her?

Competing Opinions

Perspective #1: Learning language from birth is easier than at any other time in life, and being bilingual will improve a person's cognitive abilities. Kids who speak two languages will have career and social advantages for life, and they'll be better able to appreciate other cultures. For some families it's an important connection to their own cultural heritage and identity. Why wait to offer all of the benefits that come with being bilingual? Start right away!

Perspective #2: Exposing babies to two languages while they're learning to talk might confuse them, keeping them from learning the fundamentals of either language properly. What if they mix up the words? And isn't there a chance that it could delay their speech? Of course it's an advantage in life to speak more than one language, but maybe it's better to wait before moving toward bilingualism.

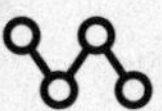

What the Science Says

RESEARCH SHOWS THAT babies growing up in bilingual homes can listen to two languages without becoming confused or experiencing a delay. They hit expected language milestones and follow roughly the same schedule as children raised in monolingual homes. Beyond that, research has shown that babies in a bilingual setting demonstrate improved cognitive and problem-solving abilities—such as stronger executive functioning and an increased ability to think about language itself (what are known as metalinguistic skills)—both as children and across the life span.

The advantages don't stop with cognitive skills. One study found that babies as young as six months demonstrated advantages in the development of attention when raised in bilingual homes. Research has shown as well that even as the child grows up and begins aging, bilingualism can protect against some of the effects of cognitive decline and Alzheimer's.

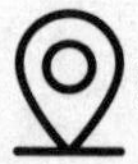

The Bottom Line

IF YOURS IS a bilingual home and you have the ability to offer both languages to your child, there are all kinds of good data about the cognitive and social benefits to suggest you should do it. If you don't have the bonus of someone at home who speaks another language, don't feel pressure to rush your baby into language lessons. There will be time later in childhood, or even once they're out of school, to learn another language.

On a Personal Note

SAD TO SAY, I'm not bilingual, and neither is my husband. But we don't have to view this as a tragedy for our kids. Short of a time machine situation where I go back and decide to date and fall in love with only multilingual people who can teach my future children a second (or third) language, there isn't much I can do about this.

Sometimes too much parenting information can feel like a curse—it can make us a bit neurotic about doing "the absolute best" for our babies. When my firstborn was six months old, I read that even at that young age, the brain was primed and ready to learn multiple languages, and that the circuitry he wasn't using for language had already begun to wither. I kind of freaked out, thinking about the missed opportunity. Soon after, when

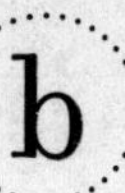

he was totally disinterested in the expensive multiple-language talking-box-cube-thing I bought because *I had to have it for him,* I actually said out loud, "Now he'll never speak Mandarin without an accent!" Fortunately, my husband didn't let me see his eyes rolling as he smiled and said, "He may turn out OK anyway."

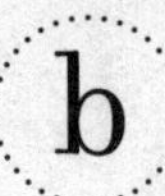

Bottles and BPA

Should you be concerned about the chemical bisphenol A (BPA) in your baby bottles, sippy cups, and containers?

Competing Opinions

Perspective #1: Since BPA is no longer contained in baby bottles, sippy cups, and infant formula packaging, plastic bottles shouldn't be a concern.

Perspective #2: Though BPA is no longer permissible in plastic baby products, those containers are best avoided because other harmful chemicals may still leach from them.

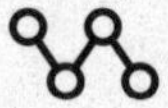

What the Science Says

BPA IS USED to make certain drink and food containers. It hardens plastic, and it's an ingredient in the lining of cans, preventing rust and offering a barrier to keep bacteria from contaminating foods. But because low levels of the chemical can leach out of the containers and into the food or beverages they house, there has long been concern about its safety. Parents and environmental groups have expressed specific concerns regarding BPA exposure and its effect on endocrine function and the reproductive system. As a result of the awareness these groups have raised, in 2009 the vast majority of manufacturers of baby bottles and sippy cups voluntarily stopped using BPA. In 2012, the American Academy of Pediatrics formally advised concerned parents to consider avoiding using clear plastic bottles that might contain BPA. In that same year, the U.S. Food and Drug Administration (FDA) officially banned BPA as a material to be used in the manufacture of baby bottles and sippy cups.

The FDA made a point, however, of emphasizing that its decision was made to boost consumer confidence and to codify officially what the industry was already doing, not because of actual safety concerns. In other words, as the FDA explained, official approval of the use of certain BPA-based materials in baby bottles, sippy cups, and infant formula packaging "is no longer necessary for the specific use of the food additive because that use has been permanently and completely abandoned." In fact, the FDA stressed in a 2018 document that it had "performed extensive research and reviewed hundreds of studies about BPA's safety" and that "current approved uses of BPA in food containers and packaging are safe." The United Kingdom's Food Standards Agency agrees, and the European Food Safety Authority likewise concludes that "BPA poses no health risk to consumers of any age group (including unborn children, infants and adolescents) at current exposure levels."

Other environmental and health organizations, including governmental agencies, aren't so sure, at least about what a safe minimum exposure level is. The U.S. Environmental Protection Agency (EPA), the National Institutes of Health (NIH), the CDC, the Endocrine Society, and the European Chemicals Agency are among those expressing at least a moderate level of concern and calling for additional research. The AAP cites evidence showing that BPA can, alarmingly, "act like estrogen in the body and potentially change the timing of puberty, decrease fertility, increase body fat, and affect the nervous and immune systems."

Because of these concerns, the AAP recommends using alternatives to plastic, like glass and stainless steel, when you can. It also advises that if you're going to use plastic bottles, avoid those with recycling codes 3, 6, and 7, unless they're labeled "biobased" or "greenware," meaning they're made from plant or biological material rather than petroleum.

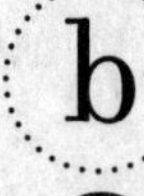

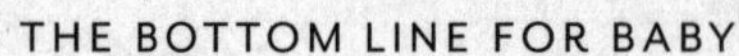

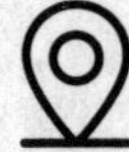

The Bottom Line

UNLESS YOU'RE USING hand-me-down bottles or sippy cups, you don't have to worry about BPA since it was banned in these products in 2012. But because the jury on the science of how much BPA is "safe" is still very much out, your best bet is to avoid plastic products labeled with recycling codes 3, 6, and 7. We can't say for sure at this point what risks BPA presents, so until we know, err on the safer side and find ways to avoid it.

Breastfeeding vs. Formula-Feeding

The benefits of breastfeeding early on are well established. The AAP goes so far as to say that because of "the documented short- and long-term medical and neurodevelopmental advantages of breastfeeding, infant nutrition should be considered a public health issue and not only a lifestyle choice." However, despite the satisfaction experienced by some mothers and babies during breastfeeding, it's not always the right choice, or even an option, for everyone. Personal preferences, medical issues, and life circumstances might lead a person to consider formula-feeding instead, or to supplement breast milk. What are the issues at stake?

Competing Opinions

Perspective #1: There are several important benefits that come with breastfeeding. For one thing, the skin-to-skin contact creates a bonding experience that's unique to the mother-child relationship. In addition, it's cheaper and more convenient than formula-feeding. And because breast milk provides a variety of tastes (having to do with what the mother has recently eaten herself), breastfeeding prepares babies to more easily accept solid foods. But the biggest benefit of breastfeeding is related to health. Breast milk boosts immunity in a way that store-bought formulas don't. What's more, breastfeeding promotes lifelong health for the baby and reduces the chances of certain cancers, diabetes, and other diseases for the mother. On top of all that, a mom who is nursing is burning calories, helping her return to her pre-pregnancy weight.

Perspective #2: While there are clearly benefits, breastfeeding is not always easy, realistic, or even possible. And the claims made by proponents of breastfeeding are sometimes overblown. The evidence isn't actually that strong that breastfeeding offers significant cognitive benefits for children. What's more, commercial formulas contain some vitamins—like vitamin D—that breastfed babies often lack and therefore have to get from supplements. And when you're formula-feeding at consistent intervals, you'll be able to more easily monitor whether your baby is getting enough to eat.

Moreover, convenience is no small factor. Going the formula route allows someone else to feed your baby at times, meaning that the child will have that many more people in her life—grandparents, siblings, aunts, uncles, sitters, and of course your partner—that she's bonding with. Furthermore, formula-fed babies sleep for longer stretches than breastfed babies. Both of those reasons also allow extra minutes for self-care, which can allow you to be a better mother.

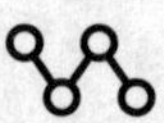

What the Science Says

RESEARCH IS CLEAR about the health benefits that breastfeeding offers. That's why the AAP recommends exclusive breastfeeding for the first six months after birth, and breastfeeding in combination with solid foods until at least age one. The WHO and UNICEF go a step further, currently recommending exclusive breastfeeding for six months and continued breastfeeding up to two years of age and beyond if possible. (See "Extended Breastfeeding" for details.)

Breast milk contains a healthy balance of nutrients and boosts the infant's immune system. It contains protein, lactose, and fats and can be more easily digested than formula, resulting in fewer bouts of diarrhea or constipation. It can also lower the risk of a long list of short- and long-term health problems for the infant, including ear infections, asthma, eczema, and respiratory infections. What may surprise you is that breastfeeding is also correlated with important benefits to the mother as well, including a lower risk of high blood pressure, type 2 diabetes, and breast and ovarian cancers.

All that said, other factors need to be considered. For example, while breast milk naturally contains important vitamins and minerals important for a newborn's healthy development, it doesn't contain enough vitamin D, which helps the body absorb calcium and phosphorus, nutrients vital for building strong bones. The AAP recommends that infants who are being breastfed (or partially breastfed) receive vitamin D supplements beginning in the first few days of life.

Keep in mind, too, that while some may vilify the use of formula instead of nursing, there are times when it actually promotes health. A recent study showed that when babies experience significant weight loss while waiting for a mother's milk to come in, early use of a limited amount of formula can offer a viable solution, keeping the babies from having to stay at the hospital or be readmitted, and the limited use of formula doesn't seem to interfere with the later success of breastfeeding.

In addition, lifestyle and life opportunities can play a big role in the decision to use formula. Some mothers simply don't have the opportunity to nurse their babies throughout the day. They might work or be in school, and there might be financial barriers that keep them from renting or purchasing a pump they would need to keep up their milk supply.

There are also rare situations in which breastfeeding isn't recommended. Broadly speaking, these exceptions occur when the mother is infected with certain viruses (such as HIV or Ebola), or when she is using certain illicit street drugs such as PCP or cocaine. Likewise, mothers should temporarily suspend breastfeeding when taking certain medications, although most medicines have little or no effect on the health of an infant. (See "Medications and Breastfeeding" for a fuller explanation.) As always, if you're not sure whether it's safe to breastfeed your baby, communicate with your physician, who should be weighing each situation on a case-by-case basis.

Regarding the claim that breastfeeding leads to higher IQ scores, there is a fair amount of debate in the scientific literature. Evidence does seem to point, though, to slightly improved cognitive benefits for children who were breastfed.

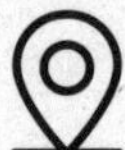

The Bottom Line

ALL MEDICAL AND health organizations recommend breastfeeding as the best option for feeding newborns and young babies. The science is clear that breastfeeding is optimal in many ways. If you have the option of nursing, do it. That being said, the decision about how to feed your child is a personal and multifaceted one, and only you, along with your doctor and your partner, if applicable, can decide what's best for your situation.

This decision is often surrounded by intense emotions. Mothers who don't nurse may experience guilt or feel shamed by others. We should keep in mind that some women *want* to nurse but can't for various reasons. Maybe they've been impacted by medical challenges like inverted nipples or even cancer. Or they might be experiencing the exhausting and frustrating problem of low milk supply, which means they end up nursing or pumping almost around the clock, often only to get very little in return. An obstacle like that, especially when combined with all the other challenges associated with parenting an infant, can take over a person's life, both physically and logistically. What's more, choosing *not* to nurse might help some mothers better meet the all-encompassing needs of their babies.

For many moms, it's not either-or. Some introduce formula for reasons related to milk supply, work schedule, caring for other children, et cetera, and still choose to breastfeed when they can, such as first thing in the morning and/or at night. This hybrid approach may work better for some, giving their babies some of the benefits of nursing while offering the additional benefit of helping mothers stick with nursing longer.

Whatever the situation, and whatever individual mothers decide for whatever reasons, we can all support one another as we each choose what's best for our families. Being unkind, harsh, and judgmental helps no one, and it rarely changes people's minds anyway. There are numerous reasons that breastfeeding is recommended by health authorities and experts around the world. But many factors should be considered in making the decision about breast milk versus formula, so if your situation or preferences lead you to use formula, you can rest assured that there are plenty of other ways to nurture your baby, both physically and emotionally.

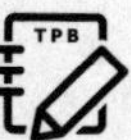

On a Personal Note

WHEN I HAD my first child, I was truly shocked to find breastfeeding so difficult. I thought it was supposed to be easy and "natural." But I was filled with confusion and questions: Was I doing it right? Was my baby doing what he was supposed to do? Was he getting enough milk? Should it hurt so much? Question after question.

We were living in rural Texas at the time, and there were no lactation consultants within seventy-five miles of us. Fortunately, I had a friend who had had a baby a year earlier, and she gave me good advice. She said that my son and I were simply learning together, and that we should just stick with it for two more weeks and see how things were going then. It was good assurance, and she was right in my case. Soon we were figuring things out, and within a few weeks my baby and I hit our stride together. Pretty quickly, then, I came to love nursing.

However, this is one of the areas where I made mistakes by being too rigid in my adherence to research. After the birth of my youngest son, the delivery nurses recommended that I temporarily supplement with formula because my milk hadn't come in yet. My son was jaundiced, and they recommended more fluids in order to flush his system. But this was my third child, and I refused to supplement. I was (and am) a huge fan of breastfeeding, I had already nursed two babies, and I was confident my milk would come in soon. It didn't, though, at least not soon enough, and my son had to return to the hospital for a few days. He was soon fine, but if I had been a bit more flexible, we likely could have avoided the whole, miserable ordeal and remained at home, comfortable, finding our way together. Instead, he was lying in a phototherapy box, and I was being told I couldn't hold him nearly as much as I wanted.

And it wasn't just flexibility I needed. I was actually missing information. If I'd known the research showing that limited supplementation with formula in the early days in cases like ours is unlikely to interfere with breastfeeding, then I could have made a better and more informed decision. In the end, it wasn't that I shouldn't have honored my commitment to what I believed regarding breastfeeding. I just needed more flexibility, and more information.

Bug Spray

DEET is a chemical in many commercial insect repellents. It protects us from bugs not by killing them but by repelling them so they won't land on our skin at all. DEET has been proven to be very effective. But is it safe for babies?

Competing Opinions

Perspective #1: Insect repellents these days are tested by governmental oversight agencies to ensure their safety. They'll keep your baby from being bitten by bugs that can cause disease or irritations.

Perspective #2: Bug sprays rely on potentially dangerous chemicals that can sink into a baby's delicate skin. It's much better to cover babies with protective clothes. Keep them indoors if necessary rather than risk chemicals seeping into their bloodstream.

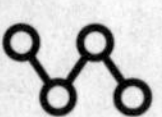

What the Science Says

FOR YEARS NOW the science has been clear on insect repellents, especially those containing DEET, or what's referred to in chemistry as N,N-diethyl-meta-toluamide. Despite 25 percent of Americans saying they avoid bug sprays containing DEET, there's not much of a debate anymore, and the scientific literature paints a clear picture: as long as it's used as directed, DEET is safe. Numerous findings support this position. Some scientists even refer to DEET as the gold standard of insect repellents.

You may have heard about findings linking DEET with seizures among children. However, a detailed review of the available research found only ten reports of seizures in children following application to the skin since DEET became available in the 1950s, and determined that none of these

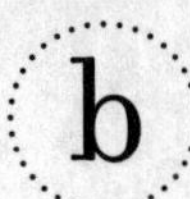

reports had been published since 1992. The authors of the study point out as well that since seizure disorders occur in 3 percent to 5 percent of children, "it would not be surprising to see an association just by chance in some cases." In other words, seizures are not significantly associated with DEET, according to the research.

Over the last couple of decades, opinions within the scientific community have generally coalesced around one primary position: that DEET is safe for both adults and children. The key exception is newborn babies under two months. Several groups of authorities caution against using insect repellent at this young and vulnerable age. Aside from that one caveat, the harmlessness of DEET when used as directed has been recognized by the CDC, the AAP, the EPA, and the U.S. Department of Health and Human Services Agency for Toxic Substances and Disease Registry.

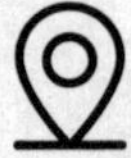

The Bottom Line

IF YOUR BABY is younger than two months, avoid insect repellents altogether. Instead, just use clothing as a barrier or mosquito netting over your stroller if you need protection. But once your child is older than two months, you can feel free to use products containing DEET—as long as you follow the directions and precautions on the bottle.

Car Seats

Some critics have cast doubt on the effectiveness of car seats in saving the lives of children. Are these doubts legitimate?

Competing Opinions

Perspective #1: Regardless of cost and inconvenience, all parents should carefully follow the guidelines for properly installing and using an age- and size-appropriate car seat to ensure children's safety.

Perspective #2: Rigid guidelines for the purchase, installation, and use of child car seats are confusing to understand and expensive to follow, and the seats may not even be as safe as people claim.

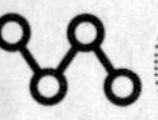

What the Science Says

WHILE THERE HAS been some debate about the overall effectiveness of car seats over the last fifteen years, none of it has revolved around a baby's first year of life. There are no credible opponents of or arguments against placing an infant in a rear-facing car seat. Holding a baby on your lap in a car or putting an infant in a forward-facing car seat is dangerous; strapping your baby into a rear-facing infant seat can save her life.

One relevant—and important—factor that the research does highlight, however, is that the vast majority of parents do not install and use infant car seats correctly. One recent study looked at 291 families as they left the newborn unit of a hospital and found that 95 percent of car seats were misused, in terms of either positioning or installation. What the authors of the study called "serious misuse" occurred in 91 percent of cases. Other studies have drawn similar conclusions, varying in specific percentages but supporting the finding that the way parents use or install infant car seats is clearly a widespread problem.

Typically, errors in usage occur regarding where parents place the seat, how tightly it's anchored into the car, the angle at which it's installed, how the baby is buckled into the seat, and whether the car seat has lost its structural integrity.

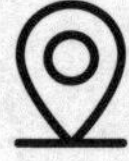

The Bottom Line

AS A PARENT, your very first job is to keep your child safe. Placing your baby in a car seat every time he's in a vehicle is your legal responsibility. Take care as well to properly install the car seat and to position your infant correctly, following all guidelines, to offer the most protection. If you'd like some assistance, there's plenty of online help, and most communities have certified car seat safety technicians who provide free installation and usage safety checks.

On a Personal Note

I WAS A bit of a control freak when it came to anyone else, other than a few people who I knew were as conscientious as I was, buckling my babies into their car seats. There were uncomfortable moments when I went back to double-check someone else's work, but if they thought I was being neurotic, that was fine with me. I felt better knowing I was reducing the risks as much as I could for my babies. As long as you're being rational, don't worry about committing to whatever you feel is helpful to protect your baby, even if others think you're over the top.

Circumcision

Circumcision is an optional procedure for infant males to surgically remove the foreskin that covers the tip (glans) of the penis. The practice is common in the United States, but much less so in other parts of the world. For parents from traditions or religious groups where boys are customarily circumcised, there may not be much of a dilemma. Most other U.S. parents will wade into a debate that can become contentious at times, and parents may find themselves conflicted as well.

Competing Opinions

Perspective #1: Circumcision comes with risks, and it just doesn't make sense to gamble with the health or physical integrity of a newborn, especially with what is essentially an elective surgery on a "private" part of the body. Aside from the avoidable, unnecessary pain to the baby boy, the penis can become irritated and even injured. Excessive bleeding and infection are possibilities as well.

Beyond the pain and risk of injury, a key reason not to circumcise is that the foreskin is a normal, healthy part of a boy's body, just like the female foreskin (clitoral hood) is a normal and healthy part of a girl's body. It's a fairly drastic step to remove that part of a child's genitalia. When a boy gets older he might decide on the procedure for himself, but circumcising an infant entails having parents decide what to do with their son's body. He should have an open future. He should have the right to make an informed decision for himself once he's old enough.

Perspective #2: The main reasons to circumcise a baby boy are related to health. Circumcision slightly reduces the risk of urinary tract infections (UTIs) during the first year of life; it decreases the chance of getting some sexually transmitted infections (STIs) later in life, including HIV; and it lowers the risk of penile cancer as well as cervical cancer in female partners. Plus, if the boy doesn't get circumcised and decides to undergo the procedure later—possibly because he's been teased for not being circumcised—the potential for complications is greater, and it will be more painful and take him longer to recover.

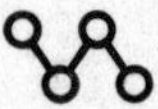 What the Science Says

RESEARCHERS ARE OFTEN split on the risks and benefits of circumcision. Let's begin with risks, the first of which is pain. Whereas previously there was a belief that newborns didn't experience pain the way adults might, it's clear that they do, and relief from that pain should be a part of any circumcision. Local anesthesia is generally effective and can consist of a penile nerve block and topical anesthetic, both during the procedure and afterward.

Another concern is infection, as is the case with any operation. However, assuming the procedure is performed properly at a hospital and parents follow post-surgical advice, such as not putting the baby in the bath until after the wound has healed, the risks are minimal. There's also the chance that further surgery might be required due to residual foreskin or what's called meatal stenosis, where the urethra is compressed, making it difficult for the child to urinate. How significant this problem is in circumcised boys ranges widely, with estimates ranging from rare (0.7 percent) to common (20 percent).

One other biological point worth addressing is the claim made by opponents that circumcision can decrease the sensitivity of the penis, meaning that sexual pleasure will be diminished later in life. This position is vigorously debated, and it is difficult at this time to draw confident conclusions regarding whether circumcision has negative effects on sexual function, sensitivity, or pleasure. Those are the primary risks that come with circumcision, although opponents of circumcision point out that the risks of the practice are still understudied.

As for the benefits, research has found a lower rate of UTIs among circumcised males. One study found that over their lifetime, one in three uncircumcised boys will get a urinary tract infection, compared with one in twelve circumcised boys. However, a recent review by the Canadian Urological Association states that the evidence of circumcision-related decreases in UTIs is insufficient to recommend universal circumcision, and opponents argue that since UTIs are minor and easily treated with antibiotics, they should not be considered as significant factors in the decision. Research has also demonstrated that circumcised males are at a lower risk of getting HIV and other STIs from an infected female partner, but these studies have been performed in Africa, and questions have been raised regarding their applicability outside of that geographical and cultural context. And evidence shows that circumcision decreases the odds of developing penile cancer. Again, though, there is debate regarding whether the risk of that cancer is great enough to be considered a significant factor.

Based on analysis of these issues, the AAP declared in a 2012 statement that the benefits of circumcision outweigh the risks, and the CDC supports that position. Both, though, stop short of recommending the procedure across the board, as do the Canadian Paediatric Society and the Canadian Urological Association. It's worth noting, too, that certain health organizations around the world disagree with the AAP statement, and a group of mostly European doctors has criticized it, pointing to what it calls cultural bias on the part of the AAP task force. It's also noteworthy that the AAP has allowed its 2012 statement to expire after the five-year mark and has so far opted not to reaffirm it.

While this book focuses more on research studies, I would be remiss if I didn't mention that a key aspect of the debate surrounding circumcision involves examining the issue from an ethical perspective. In 2019 more than ninety ethicists and scholars published an article arguing that, as one of the authors put it, "children of all sexes and genders have a right to be protected from genital cutting that isn't medically necessary."

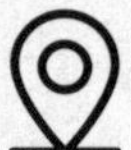

The Bottom Line

BOTH PROPONENTS AND opponents claim that the debate about circumcision is over. It clearly isn't. Increasingly, medical authorities (especially those outside the United States) are concluding that circumcision can't be justified based on any health benefits it offers. But authors in the field still strongly disagree as to whether that's the case. If you have misgivings about the practice for your child, you'll find no shortage of support in the available evidence. Likewise, though, if you're already committed to circumcising your baby, you can also find evidence that supports your decision and authorities who agree with you.

This is one example of the many parenting (and non-parenting) decisions where we can be driven more by our values, beliefs, tradition, emotions, preconceptions, and culture than by information and facts. In other words, if we already hold a particular position, then we might tend to pay attention to and reassure ourselves with the rational scientific data that bolster our view. If you're conflicted but feel like you want your son to "look like his dad" or "follow family tradition," then you're more likely to find the data and arguments on the health benefits of circumcision more compelling, and the claims about the risks or concerns less significant. On the other hand, if you're conflicted but it really bothers you that a doctor is going to remove a healthy part of your child's body and cause unnecessary pain, then you may be more likely to find the data and arguments on the risks of circumcision more compelling, and the evidence on the benefits minimal.

I would love to give you clear-cut advice based on the science, but in this case, the decision is up to you. In conversation with your pediatrician, weigh the risks and benefits for your child, then take into account other issues including culture, religion, premature birth, family medical history, personal preference and values, and any ethical and human rights concerns you may have. All of these factors can lead you to the best decision you can make for your son.

C

Co-sleeping

Should you let your infant share your bed? Or are the risks—primarily SIDS—so great that the practice should be avoided?

Competing Opinions

Perspective #1: Co-sleeping increases the chance of your child being smothered inadvertently (by you or by the covers) and increases the risk of sudden infant death syndrome (SIDS) or one of the other types of sudden unexpected infant death (SUID). In 2016, the AAP even released a new policy statement that bed-sharing should definitely not take place for the first six months, and preferably not until the baby turns one. Also, bed-sharing often leads to less overall sleep for both child and parent, at a time when meaningful rest is both crucial and hard to come by. Plus, once your child gets used to sleeping with you, it can be hard to get him to stop. It's best not to co-sleep with your baby.

Perspective #2: While there are certain risks that come with co-sleeping, the rewards far outweigh them. Parents all over the world sleep with their babies. For many parents there's a strong instinctual drive to sleep next to their newborn, and their family and cultural traditions support that drive. Plus, having the baby sleep close to the parent promotes bonding and more effective breastfeeding, both of which are important developmental processes. And while some claim bed-sharing prevents sleep for both baby and parent, many parents swear that it actually promotes it, since the baby can be more easily, quickly, and conveniently soothed when she wakes during the night. As for getting babies to sleep in their own bed when the time comes, there are plenty of ways to make that transition when it's time. As long as careful safety precautions are taken, co-sleeping can be rewarding and beneficial for both parent and child.

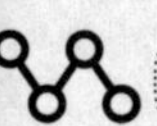

What the Science Says

DESPITE THE AAP'S warning against it, co-sleeping has quadrupled in U.S. homes in the last twenty-five years as families have increasingly valued parent-child bonding. The AAP position, understandably, as it seeks to keep babies as safe as possible, appears to emerge from an abundance of caution, since the science isn't quite definitive on the issue. For example, some studies correlating SIDS and bed-sharing have failed to take into account the type of sleeping environment, such as the surface the baby was sleeping on at the time. (Soft cushions are much less safe than a firm mattress.) As of this writing, almost no reliable data exists from rigorous studies that have examined the question while considering sleeping surface. The small amounts of data that do exist suggest that after three months of age, there is little or no additional risk of SIDS for babies who share their parents' bed, if precautions are followed. For younger newborns, the danger appears to increase, but still can be relatively insignificant for babies when there are no risk factors present. However, and this is important, if certain risk factors do exist—if parents drink or smoke or use drugs, or if the child was born premature or with other health issues, or if caregivers are not following safe co-sleeping guidelines—the concern is greater, and it's not safe to co-sleep. (Smoking seems to correlate especially strongly with the risk of SIDS.)

Several studies have also shown that co-sleeping correlates with important positive outcomes, such as better sleep, more stable infant heart rates, improved parent-child bonding, mutual soothing, and more effective and consistent breastfeeding. That being said, negative effects beyond the risk of SIDS have been found as well. A recent study showed that "maternal distress" sometimes correlates with co-sleeping beyond six months, in that mothers who share either a room or a bed with their infants are more likely to feel depressed and criticized for their decision.

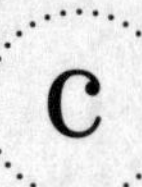

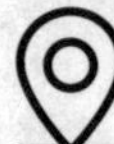

The Bottom Line

SIDS AND SUID are valid concerns when it comes to co-sleeping, and it's likely safest not to have your young infant in the bed while you sleep. But the science isn't quite as clear as many believe, partly because the research typically hasn't looked at enough specifics to parse out which co-sleeping practices are safe and which are not, so they often lead to generalized conclusions or recommendations that co-sleeping is "safe" or "not safe." My best understanding of the research is that co-sleeping can be safe or unsafe, depending on *how* you do it and what risk factors are present. For example, it's actually less likely, statistically speaking, that a typically healthy baby will die of SIDS than be hit by lightning at some point in his life. Still, it's a risk, one with unthinkable consequences. If, based on your values, instincts, traditions, and situation, you decide to co-sleep, you can do it in safer ways or in unsafe ways, so it's very important that you follow up-to-date safety guidelines and discuss the decision with your pediatrician.

For example, you should never co-sleep in a recliner or on a sofa or beanbag or anything of the sort. Also, you shouldn't co-sleep, under any circumstances, if you or anyone else in the bed has been drinking, using drugs or medications that have a sedative effect, or if you or anyone else in the house smokes. Likewise, you should follow the standard advice for all babies, including making sure they're sleeping on their back, are wearing light clothes, and are not surrounded by bulky, soft bedding or stuffed animals. Similarly, some authorities recommend that you avoid co-sleeping if you aren't breastfeeding, primarily because your biological rhythms aren't as "synced up" with your child in that case. If you do decide to share a bed, make sure that you've created the safest possible environment by minimizing pillows and blankets, removing side rails that could entrap the baby, not having other children in the bed, assuming a safer co-sleeping position, and so on. This paragraph isn't meant to be fully comprehensive regarding every precaution. If you choose to co-sleep, search online for the latest information from reputable sources and talk to your pediatrician, so you can mitigate the risk and make sleeping with your infant safer.

An even safer, hybrid solution that offers many of the benefits and less of the risks, and that is preferred by many parents, is to co-sleep on separate surfaces. You can use a "co-sleeper," a bassinet that hooks onto your bed and allows your baby to sleep right next to you but sidesteps many of the dangers described above, or you can place the crib near your bed. If you want the potential benefits that come with co-sleeping but want to be as safe as possible, this is a great solution.

On a Personal Note

I LOVED USING a co-sleeper bassinet with all of my infants the first couple of months. I felt better having them close to me so that anytime I woke, I could check on them, change them if necessary, nurse them, and then put them back to sleep more easily. It also made it easier to pull our sons into our bed to hold them, or for my husband and me to chat while the baby was there with us and happy, just hanging out, especially in the early days when I was recovering from delivery. It was easy to see that our babies were happiest, felt safest, and rarely cried when they were physically close to us. And, I felt safer having them co-sleep on a separate surface, rather than in the bed.

Then when the babies outgrew the co-sleeper, or when I was ready for them to move out of the room, which was at different ages for each of our boys, I liked having them in the crib in their own room, which the kids shared with one another. I found that I slept much better knowing they were safe, and that I didn't wake every time my baby made a noise or moved. Since I was nursing and did a lot of babywearing, I also needed the physical break at night so that I could be ready to do it again the next day.

The claim that parents should avoid co-sleeping because the baby will never learn to sleep in their own bed holds little weight for me. The same goes for the worry that the presence of a child in the family bed for a while will interfere with the couple's sex life. Kids do learn to sleep in their own bed, and there are plenty of ways to maintain relational intimacy for the couple.

Fear-based, future-focused parenting often keeps us from fully attuning to who our children are at a particular point in their development, and it ignores how much things change in development month to month and even week to week. Those parental worries just aren't rational when we understand development. Kids need different things from us at different times. The concern that letting a child sleep in your room will mean they won't ever learn to sleep by themselves is as silly as saying, "If you let them use a diaper they won't ever learn to use the toilet." Each child is different, and each parent is different, and the reason our kids like to sleep near us is because it helps them feel safe, and it feels good to them. A lot of adults prefer not to sleep alone as well! This makes sense. Sleep, from a survival standpoint, is a very vulnerable time, and we're less vulnerable if there are others in close proximity to alert and wake us for safety and protection.

As for the sex argument, if there's a kid sleeping in your room, then have sex somewhere else in the house. Some creativity may be required, but a little novelty might come in handy right now as well!

Daycare or Nanny?

If you've decided you won't be staying at home with your baby, how do you decide between a nanny and another kind of daycare?

Competing Opinions

Perspective #1: Infants and young children do best when one person gives them the care and attention they require. Not everyone can afford a nanny, obviously, but if you can find someone to be a consistent presence in your child's life, that will come with all kinds of advantages. The main benefit is that your child will have an additional primary attachment figure she knows she can count on when you're not there, and her needs will be tended to consistently.

Perspective #2: What matters most is quality. If you can find a good daycare center near you, that's better than having a nanny who may or may not be adequately focused on the needs of your child. Plus, daycare centers have some accountability, since they have to be certified and provide a certain amount of education for the caregivers. Nannies might not even be trained in CPR, much less the basics of supportive child rearing. Also, daycare provides socialization opportunities that can benefit babies' social and emotional development.

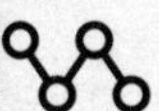

What the Science Says

IT'S REALLY DIFFICULT to discuss what the science says about choosing a nanny as opposed to a daycare center. There is ample scientific literature comparing non-parental childcare with stay-at-home parents. But direct data demonstrating the nanny-daycare difference is much harder to come by.

One experiment, a French study published in 2018, compared children ranging in age from birth to three years in the care of one non-parental caregiver to those in center-based childcare. These children were in a cohort of 1,428 children who were followed from pregnancy to eight years of age. The study concluded that kids in the daycare centers were more likely to experience emotional, relational, and social success than those looked after by a single non-parental caregiver and to exhibit fewer conduct problems. There were plenty of variables at play—for example, girls and children from families with a higher socioeconomic status reaped more benefits than boys and kids from lower-socioeconomic-status families—but overall, the childcare centers appeared to help kids reduce future social and emotional difficulties. However, the study's conclusion emphasized that "high-quality" childcare is what produces the most advantageous outcomes. (More about that later.)

Most of the research on this subject focuses less on the "daycare or nanny" question, and more on the difference between kids being cared for in a "formal" arrangement (like childcare centers, Head Start, and pre-kindergarten), on one hand, and in an "informal" arrangement (like home-based care outside a child's home, or home-based care in the child's home by a nanny, babysitter, or unpaid family member), on the other. Generally speaking, formal childcare produces more positive outcomes than informal care in terms of cognition and behavior. A significant reason for these differences is the regulatory oversight formal childcare centers are subject to. As one study put it, "Children enrolled in formal care experience higher quality with respect to all four categories we considered: caregiver characteristics, safety, activities, and observed quality. . . . [W]e also note that quality is highest in arrangements subject to the most stringent regulations."

I could point to many other studies that support these conclusions, but the problem is that these investigations aren't precisely focused on our question here. For one thing, they're broad, focusing on informal childcare in general, rather than just non-parental caregivers or nannies. In addition, the studies are often looking at preschoolers and older kids, not just babies.

In the absence of a clear and wide body of scientific literature to direct us, I can offer two key research-based principles to help guide you. First of all, what babies get from their families is crucial. Speaking generally, the research is clear that the most important factor when it comes to what's best for babies down the road, in terms of behavior, health, and cognition, is not the *type* of care they receive—from a childcare center, nanny, preschool, relative, or even parent—but what the home experience is like. Much more important than where kids receive care is the degree to which they receive love, warmth, responsiveness, cognitive stimulation, and so on when they're at home. In other words, *where* they are cared for matters less than *how* they are cared for in their home environment by their parents and families.

The other key principle is not exactly shocking: quality matters. A lot. Study after study supports what you already know, that early childhood experiences shape kids and impact who they become, so the quality of those experiences matters profoundly. And I'm afraid that there's plenty of research demonstrating how inconsistent that quality is when it comes to childcare of all kinds.

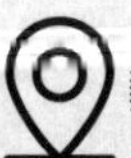

The Bottom Line

WHAT MATTERS MORE than anything is that you provide a consistent, loving, nurturing, enriching home environment, and that whatever childcare decision you make, you make it with quality in mind. Studies do seem to support the idea that formal daycare provides more consistent quality than informal childcare like what nannies and relatives might offer, but those conclusions are drawn from a wide range of situations. There's no question that if you have access to and can afford a caring, high-quality nanny, that's preferable to a third-rate childcare center. And the opposite is true as well, of course: a quality daycare center is definitely preferable to a nanny you can't count on. Finally, try to obtain childcare that will provide as little turnover as possible when it comes to the person or people your child learns to depend on.

Daycare or Stay at Home?

What's involved in deciding whether to stay at home with the kids as opposed to going back to work? Are there benefits of one over the other?

Competing Opinions

Perspective #1: If you have the means and the desire to stay home with your kids, that's the best thing you can do for them. It shows them that you've made them a priority and gives you the opportunity to be the most consistent and influential presence in their lives. This is the best way to ensure that your child is getting quality care, and you won't miss out on important moments.

Perspective #2: There are plenty of good reasons for a parent of small children to work. You might have the kind of job you love and find fulfilling or meaningful, or you might simply need the income. Maybe you like the idea of having your kids see you contribute in this way, doing important work in the world, or maybe you find that it makes you a better parent since you can return home eager to be with them, with less parental burnout. Or maybe you just want to.

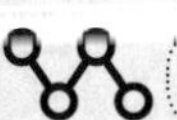

What the Science Says

FIRST OF ALL, the way it's usually discussed—whether to work or stay home to raise the kids—presents a false dichotomy that oversimplifies a personal, complicated, and often difficult decision. For one thing, as many people have noted through the years, it's not fair or accurate to imply that stay-at-home parents (SAHPs) aren't "working"; being a SAHP can be one of the most demanding and arduous jobs around, with "bosses" (babies) who can be ruthless and narcissistic! It's also not fair or accurate to say that working parents aren't spending a lot of time with their children. Even though they're working, they're often spending more time overall with their kids than parents did decades ago.

What's more, for many parents, their finances and/or life situation mean that staying at home with kids simply isn't a good option. Others make the opposite decision, pausing their careers because they can't afford the high cost of quality childcare or because they can't find an available, quality option that makes them comfortable.

A probably infinite number of other variables are at play as well. Some parents are married, and some are single. Some have grandparents who can step up and provide quality care, while others have grandparents who are willing but who won't provide truly positive, quality care. Some enjoy robust networks of friends and communities who support one another, while some have only a small network of support, if that. Some have money, and some are struggling to get by. Plus, some parents want to stay at home more when the kids are little, then return to work; some want to work part-time; some want to work from home. Technology has also changed the workforce in many fields, allowing parents to work remotely or more flexibly, allowing them opportunities to be with their babies more. Many families find some combination of working outside the home and caring for the baby that changes over time. The issues, and the dynamics at play, are complex, messy, multidimensional, and fluid.

Rather than reduce this multifaceted challenge to a straightforward, two-sided dilemma about working versus staying home with the kids, we should help parents gather as much credible information as they can and then let them do their best in their particular situations. Some will be fortunate enough to be able to choose their work-parenting balance, while others don't have that luxury at all. For virtually all families, though, whatever the ultimate outcome, it will mean making sacrifices and experiencing regrets as well as creating all kinds of joy and fulfillment, all while having to continually revisit questions about an always evolving set of circumstances and revise their plans depending on changing circumstances.

The good news is that a huge amount of research has been published over the last few decades concerning "early maternal employment" (EME), defined as mothers working during a child's first three years, focusing on its effect on children's health, behavior, social development, academics, cognitive abilities, and so on. (By the way, some of the studies discussed here have examined parents in general, but most have looked at mothers in particular. There are plenty of times when moms and dads experience certain parenting realities similarly, and we can all be grateful for the evolving societal attitudes regarding fathers and caregiving. But based on the research, this particular question represents one of those moments where gender likely matters, and women's experiences are situationally unique. I'll therefore be specific when investigators have focused on mothers rather than fathers.)

The bad news is that summaries of these various studies consistently declare the overall takeaway from the science to be that the findings are "complicated," "mixed," and "competing"—and therefore difficult to apply toward simple or confident conclusions. As one set of investigators put it, "Over the years, research on maternal employment and children's achievement has been consistent only in producing mixed results."

Take children's cognition and behavior, for example. How are they affected by having a working mother? Well, some studies indicate that the correlation can be positive, and some indicate that it's negative. Further complicating the issue is that still other studies, when looking at details of the mother's work (like the nature of her job or the age of the child), report both positive *and* negative results. And one meta-analysis in 2008 looked at sixty-eight different studies and eventually concluded that there's essentially no significant association between maternal employment and what they called "children's achievement." Generally speaking, though, various summaries of the research suggest that daycare is often associated with better cognitive development and slightly worse behavior.

Conflicting results like these can be found in response to all kinds of research questions regarding EME and children's outcomes. As you might expect, strong and secure parent-child relationships are linked to improved cognitive development and behavior. Some studies have shown that EME has the potential to disrupt the formation of secure attachment. Other studies have found that attachment can be impacted more by a later return to work, once the relationship has been established, than by a mother working while the early relationship is forming. So that would lead to some parental concern about working outside the home. But a host of other studies have looked at care by people other than the mother and shown positive outcomes of various daycare options, demonstrating that quality childcare experiences are linked to better cognitive and social competencies. And yet these findings are complicated in that more time spent in childcare of poorer quality has been shown to correspond with less-sensitive overall parenting, meaning that these correlations are, again, complicated.

What about stress? Is it harder on the parents themselves when they're in the official workforce or when they're raising kids at home? Well, a 2012 Gallup poll of more than sixty thousand U.S. women found that stay-at-home mothers are more likely than working moms to report depression, sadness, and anger. But guess what other studies show? Yep. Mothers who are working full-time while raising a child experience significantly higher stress levels, with their biological markers showing signs of even higher levels of stress when there's a second child.

It's far outside the scope of this book to go into all of the other issues that research explores when it comes to parents' decision about working outside the home. But you get the picture. It's hard to draw clear and firm scientific conclusions because the overall evidence is often working against itself. That being said, though, we can use various overviews and meta-analyses that have looked at research on the subject and offered overarching claims regarding what it all means.

The biggest claim of all, one that I hope will make you take a big sigh of relief, is that if there are actual effects on children—either positive or negative—resulting from whether their parents work outside the home, those effects are minor. It's not that there's no difference at all. As Emily Oster puts it in her very helpful book *Cribsheet*, it looks like "the impacts of both parents working are positive (i.e., working is better) for kids from poorer families, and less positive (or even slightly negative) for children from richer families." But Oster follows up this statement by stressing that any significant effects on child development when parents work "are small or zero."

Various meta-analyses from the last few years tend to agree. The majority of studies highlight the positive outcomes associated with some sort of maternity/paternity leave and/or a consistent parental presence during a child's first year. Aside from the early stages in a baby's life, though, children of mothers who work don't seem to experience any significant consequences, either positive or negative. Another point of emphasis is the important role that family and background variables play when it comes to the question of EME. Race, culture, education, income, and other social factors can all influence the extent to which EME affects children's overall outcomes.

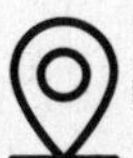

The Bottom Line

PEOPLE TALK ABOUT the "mommy wars," and there are few more emotionally charged battlefields in those confrontations than the one over the choice of whether to stay at home with the kids. It's unfortunate and unhelpful when anyone approaches the conversation with judgment rather than a desire to listen and understand. My first point of the bottom line here, then, is that I hope we can all move past our criticism of one an-

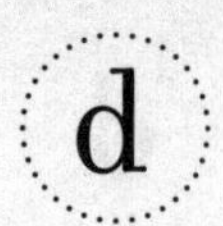

other regarding this question. Virtually all parents are doing everything they can to make the best decision possible for themselves and their family, and the more we can all support one another, the better we'll all be at raising good kids and making the world a better place.

As for a more specific bottom line regarding the science on this issue, there are a few key points throughout the research literature. One is the importance of devoted, attuned caregivers. A high-quality daycare center, where the child is loved and held and given attention, is obviously better than being at home with a parent who is constantly distracted or unable to provide for the baby's physical and emotional needs because she's overwhelmed, depressed, or resentful about her life decisions.

Other considerations include your desires, what other options you have regarding the kind and quality of care your kids will receive in your absence, and your resources, in terms of finances as well as support from friends and family members. Returning to Oster again, I like her recommendation that you break your decision down into three components: what's best for your child, what you want to do, and what the implications of your choice are for the family budget. If you do go the childcare route, make sure to pick a quality center that has a high number of caregivers so there are enough adults to care for the babies, and one that has really low turnover. The caregivers who spend a lot of time with your baby become attachment figures for the child. The good news is that babies can have several attachment figures, so that doesn't take away from how special you are to your baby, but you want to make sure that those attachment figures your baby learns to trust are stable and not a revolving door.

Research says that especially in the early months, it's highly beneficial to stay with your baby if you can work it out. Aside from that, though, there's no global, inherently right or wrong decision. Make the call that feels most right for your child, yourself, and your family, knowing that there are sacrifices and drawbacks that come with the benefits you enjoy with any decision. It won't be easy, but let your love for your child lead you to the best choice possible given your current circumstances.

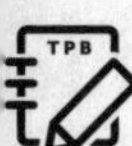

On a Personal Note

I'LL ADMIT THAT I have distinct opinions about how I think things "should" be done in my life. I'm super-conscientious (OK, I can be a control freak), and I often expect others around me to be the same way. (Yes, I'm aware that this isn't always fun for the other people.) But right or wrong, especially when it comes to my children, I have, shall we say, really strong preferences. As a new parent, those preferences were that I stay home with my kids.

From the time I was a little girl, I always wanted to be a stay-at-home mom. Most of my jobs through high school and college involved caring for children. My husband and I waited six years before we had babies because it was so important to me to stay home. By that time, my husband, Scott, had finished his graduate education and we could afford for me not to work.

So I stayed home with our baby. We planned carefully, lived frugally, got some help from our parents, and managed to scrape by financially—at least until Scott got a job in California, where my family was, and where I was eager to return. As we quickly learned, living expenses in California can be drastically different from those in rural West Texas. I remember the night Scott said to me, "This isn't working on one salary. We can't make it like this."

I responded, "But that wasn't the plan. I'm staying home with the kids." My rebuttal didn't solve our problem very well.

So I decided that if I *had* to work, I'd be a professor with family-friendly hours, summers off, holiday breaks, and the flexibility to attend recitals, pick up kids from school, and so on. I entered a PhD program, taking classes and studying when Scott could be home to watch our son. Over the course of getting my degree, I had two more babies. Creatively working our schedules, I was still able to stay home with my boys, studying in the wee hours, during naptimes, and in chunks when Scott could take the boys to the park. I was exhausted for many of those years in order to do what I really desired: to be with my kids during their waking hours.

My plans to be a professor changed along the way—I became a child and adolescent therapist and saw clients one day a week when Scott could be home with the boys. That became a passion for me, and soon I was teaching about parenting and the brain. I met and studied with Dan Siegel, and we wrote *The Whole-Brain Child,* which came out when my youngest began kindergarten. At that time I began traveling a good bit, speaking to parents, educators, and professionals, all of which led to the writing of this book. As my boys got older, I began working more, and to this day I'm still *always* trying to navigate the right balance of caregiving and working for me and for our family. I often don't start my workday until around 8:30 at night, after dinner and bedtime routines, so I'm not sure I'm balancing things well lots of days. But I don't want to miss out on time in the afternoon and evening hours when my boys are home.

While I was a stay-at-home mom, I had the luxury of a partner who could be with our boys a lot and play a big role in co-parenting, so I could study or work in spurts, or sleep a bit later when I was up late working the night before. Still, it was really hard, the way we did things. I realize that not everyone has the support or financial wherewithal to stay at home with their kids. I get it. I've been there. Whatever decisions we make about working while parenting, we're going to have to make sacrifices, and we're going to miss out on something either way. Staying at home was extremely challenging, exhausting, and, at times, maddening. I often didn't find all the menial tasks of caring for my family as rewarding or joyful as I imagined they would be. And still, I wouldn't change anything about those years I spent at home with my boys. It was the right decision for me and for our family. And then, when I started working, that was challenging as well. We do the best we can do, given our circumstances, to make the choices that work for our lives while also showing up for our kids and being there to give them what they need. And there are lots and lots of ways to do that, whether you stay home or not.

One final point here: I hope we can stop using the gendered phrase "mommy wars." I love that more dads are staying at home with their babies and young children, and playing much bigger roles in caring for their kids, thus giving families even more options to consider.

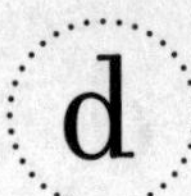

Diapers: Disposable vs. Cloth

The vast majority of American parents—by some estimates 95 percent—use disposable diapers at least sometimes for their babies. But cloth diapers offer an alternative that more and more parents turn to. Choosing between the options involves considering what's best for your baby, for you, for your family, and for the environment.

Competing Opinions

Perspective #1: Cloth diapers are better for the environment. They're cheaper in the long run, and cloth is a better material to have against an infant's delicate skin. Plus, they don't contain the chemicals present in disposable diapers that may have allergenic consequences.

Perspective #2: Disposable diapers are more convenient and sanitary. They'll keep the baby drier and less likely to suffer from diaper rash. And they're not even necessarily worse for the environment, since the washing and delivery of cloth diapers waste natural resources.

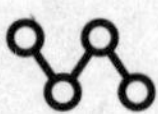

What the Science Says

THIS IS A topic where, while various sources will highlight numbers regarding environmental impact and other variables, there's not much actual research to point to. Perhaps that's why both the AAP and the EPA have remained neutral in the debate regarding cloth and disposable diapers.

There's no denying that disposable diapers impact the environment negatively. The production of the plastic and the gels that make up the diapers produces waste that must be disposed of. Then think of the packaging and marketing process—the dyes, the boxes, the delivery—and all the environmental costs that come with that. Also, the diapers are made from polypropylene, a type of plastic that is made from the nonrenewable resource petroleum and will not biodegrade under landfill conditions. Finally, the fecal contents of the diapers can end up in our groundwater.

All that said, though, cloth diapers aren't the slam dunk you'd assume, environmentally speaking. They are preferable when it comes to environmental impact, but the difference between the two options isn't as significant as you'd expect. Consider that cloth diapers are typically made from cotton, the growing of which relies on water and an inordinately heavy use of chemical fertilizers and insecticides. Then there are production costs as well as the necessity of washing them in hot water and drying them (both processes requiring energy) by the consumer. Yes, there are commercial delivery services, but the trucks create air pollution and consume resources.

What's more, additional green options are appearing each day. There are now hybrid diapers, with a cloth shell you reuse and a biodegradable liner that's safe for the sewage system and can therefore be flushed. Also, disposable diaper companies are offering chlorine-free diapers with lower levels of certain toxins, and cloth diapers are available that have been produced with organically grown, pesticide-free cotton. All of these choices, of course, raise the expense of the diapers, meaning that for many families these alternatives aren't a viable option.

Diaper rash is another factor some parents consider. Disposable diapers are thought to keep the baby drier and therefore more effectively avoid rash, but if either type of diaper is changed frequently, diaper rash can be largely prevented. One study did find that colorful dyes from disposable diapers caused an allergic reaction in a small number of children, but one of the study's authors acknowledged that the "vast majority" of children should be fine to wear the colorful diapers without incident.

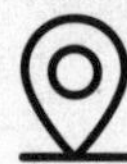

The Bottom Line

DO WHAT WORKS best for your family. The choice between disposable and cloth diapers comes down to the personal preferences of the parents. Both have advantages, and unfortunately, neither is particularly eco-friendly. For parents who can afford it and want to enjoy the convenience of disposability without the fear of saturating our landfills with additional plastic, a flushable, biodegradable liner inserted into a cloth diaper might be something to try. In any case, the most important thing to remember is to change your baby's diaper—cloth or disposable—often, to avoid rash and discomfort for your infant.

On a Personal Note

I'M A WASTE-CONSCIOUS person, and while I considered both options, disposable diapers were less expensive and more convenient for us. The truth is that by the time I got to my third baby, I just did what was easiest, and for us that was disposable.

My thinking was, "I deal with three little boys and a dog every day, and I'm touching and handling more mammalian waste than any person should have to." Seriously. I was dealing with a shockingly huge amount of bodily fluids on a moment-by-moment basis. Plus, I was so busy and showering so little that I felt like my own personal water conservation could help me justify any environmental cost of using disposable diapers.

I hesitate to officially record this next story for posterity, but here goes.

When I was pregnant with my first, I was given the acclaimed Diaper Genie, created to store soiled diapers next to the changing table until you would empty the contraption and take it to the trash. I used it a few times but then decided to return it to the store.

So as our first outing after my son was born, three weeks into our sleep deprivation and exhaustion, Scott and I made our big trip to the local Walmart. He returned the box at customer service while I held our son, glad to be out for a short time. Our newborn got hungry, so we headed home.

As I turned on the TV and sat down to nurse, an important question popped into my head. I called to my husband in the next room: "Babe, you *emptied* the Genie before you put it back in the box, right?"

Silence. Laughter. Mortification. More laughter.

I still cringe when I imagine that Genie being shelved again, someone buying it for a baby shower, and an expectant mom opening the box, right there in front of her friends and family, and finding dirty diapers inside!

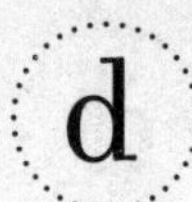

Diet and Breastfeeding

Different cultures and traditions around the world advise mothers to avoid certain foods—everything from chicken to tomatoes to anything cold—and these prescriptions can lead to unnecessary dietary restrictions and become barriers to breastfeeding. But what foods *do* affect babies, and how much should nursing moms worry about what they eat? Will eating your favorite cheesy and spicy foods cause discomfort for your nursing baby? Can you responsibly enjoy a cup of coffee or a glass of wine?

Competing Opinions

Perspective #1: Traces of what a mother eats and drinks make their way into breast milk and can affect an infant. Dairy products, alcohol, fish, caffeine, and spicy foods can all lead to allergies and/or an uncomfortable and colicky baby.

Perspective #2: Generally speaking, as long as you maintain a healthy diet, you don't need to limit what you eat while breastfeeding. Unless your baby has a negative reaction to a particular food, you can eat and drink whatever you like, including moderate amounts of fish, spicy foods, chocolate, caffeine, and alcohol.

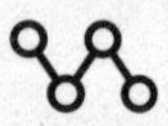

What the Science Says

AS A GENERAL rule, mothers who have developed healthy eating habits overall can continue with their normal diet while nursing. While small percentages of certain ingested foods will be transferred to breast milk and possibly even affect its smell and flavor, typical and wise intake of caffeine, spicy foods, chocolate, acidic foods, and alcohol shouldn't affect your infant. It's true that a high level of caffeine consumption could result in excessive stimulation of a baby, and more than a moderate amount of alcohol can negatively affect your child. (See the entry "Alcohol and Breastfeeding.") It's also important to keep in mind that the bodies of preterm and newborn babies are slower to break down what they take in, so caution should be exercised in those situations. But studies show that if you make healthy choices and follow nourishing, well-balanced eating habits, you don't have to worry much about your food having negative consequences for your baby.

Still, it's important to remain aware of reactions to certain foods. Just as you'd watch your baby for any additional signs of fussiness when you've had an extra cup of coffee, keep an eye out for other symptoms after you have finished, for example, a glass of milk. Cow's milk protein allergy can occur in certain infants, and its symptoms can be significantly alleviated by having the mother eliminate milk and milk products. Likewise, some breastfed infants can develop the skin allergy atopic dermatitis, and the mother's elimination of antigens from cow's milk and eggs can have a positive result. Aside from this one allergy, though, there's no strong evidence that a mother's elimination diet will result in fewer allergic reactions in her child.

Fish is another food to be educated about. It's an excellent source of proteins, vitamins, and minerals, and that can be valuable during the nursing phase, both for mother and for child. But some fish have high levels of mercury (in turn the result of what *they* eat), which is something you should limit ingestion of and exposure to when you're pregnant or breastfeeding. You'll therefore want to remain aware of how much seafood you're eating and where it comes from, since mercury can be transferred through breast milk and result in negative effects on the baby's brain and nervous system. But there are plenty of types of fish that are both nutritious and low in mercury, so if you do your homework and make good decisions, you should be able to take advantage of the many health benefits of eating fish. A general rule of thumb is that the smaller the fish, the lower the mercury content, because they are lower on the food chain and are eaten before they themselves accumulate too much mercury in their systems. Big fish eat a lot of little fish and live longer, so they tend to have a buildup of mercury in their flesh.

One other subject related to this question has to do with colic. Various studies over the years have claimed that dietary changes—for instance, cutting out cow's milk—can reduce colic. But recent meta-analyses have pointed to methodological biases and shortcomings in these studies and concluded that the evidence demonstrating the connection between colic and a mother's diet is sparse.

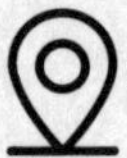

The Bottom Line

EATING A HEALTHY, diverse diet is good for both mom and baby. There are very few foods that you need to worry about, and some of your spicy favorites may even add a little flavor to your nursing baby's cuisine. Do avoid fish that can be high in mercury levels, and if you have a glass of wine, be sure to give it time (usually two hours) to clear your system before you nurse your baby. (See the entry "Alcohol and Breastfeeding.") Also, if your baby has colic, a skin reaction, or other signs of discomfort, or if you have any questions or wonder about specific circumstances for you or your infant, be sure to consult your pediatrician, as certain food eliminations may be helpful for your child.

Discipline

You may think that discipline won't be an issue for most of the first year of your baby's life. And while it's true that typical boundary-pushing and limit-setting won't come into play for several months, how you interact with and respond to your infant now can lay the foundation for how you handle behavioral issues throughout your little one's childhood. Now's the time to begin thinking about your philosophy and how you want to approach discipline with your baby.

Competing Opinions

Perspective #1: *The authoritarian approach.* Children need rules and boundaries, and they should obey them. The world isn't going to explain things to them or let them talk back or question authority; they'll be expected to understand what they're supposed to do, then do it. You shouldn't have to explain your reasons, and kids should do as you say. When they disobey, be strict. Punishment helps them learn their lesson and have a healthy fear of their parents. Within a few months you need to make sure your baby understands the meaning of the word "no."

Perspective #2: *The permissive approach.* The best way to express your love is to be warm and responsive relationally, but then take more of a hands-off approach when it comes to setting rules. Even as your baby gets older, you should worry more about communicating how much you love your child than on making her do the things you want her to do.

Perspective #3: *The authoritative approach.* Children do need limits and boundaries, but you can respect your kids enough to take the time to explain or discuss the rules you're setting up. With babies, you'll have to set limits as they get closer to one year of age, but make sure you do that in a

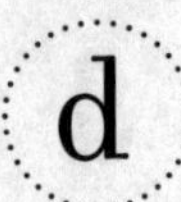

way that's warm and nurturing. When clear expectations and limits are combined with respectful feedback, connection, and nurturing love, kids will feel safe in the world. They won't just rely on adults when it comes to making good decisions, but instead will develop self-control, along with independence and inner confidence.

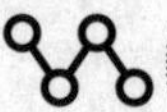

What the Science Says

THE THREE PERSPECTIVES described in the previous section represent parenting styles first formally identified by the developmental psychologist Diana Baumrind in the 1960s, and her model has had a momentous impact on the science of child rearing ever since. To this day scholars studying parenting approaches rely on the basic framework Baumrind set up more than fifty years ago.

The key idea is that there are two primary dimensions to be considered when we discuss parenting styles:

> *Connection* (which has typically been called warmth or nurture) is the degree of affection, emotional responsiveness, and attunement parents bring to their interactions with their kids.

> *Structure* (often called, unfortunately, control or demandingness) refers to the demands parents make on their children in terms of asking them to adhere to expectations and follow the rules and guidelines presented to them. You can think of parental structure as setting clear and consistent limits and boundaries.

Using these two dimensions, we can discuss different parenting styles. If a parent is high on structure and low on connection, then she's going to be more *authoritarian* in her approach. She'll strictly demand that her kids toe the line, and she'll require unquestioned obedience, often punishing them when they don't obey. Punishments may even be harsh or shaming. (See the entry "Spanking.") These high expectations will be joined with high maturity demands, and there won't be much tolerance for questioning rules and orders. Displays of affection will be fairly rare as well. This is the attitude in Perspective #1. You can see in the following image that an authoritarian parenting style is in the quadrant that's high on structure but low on connection.

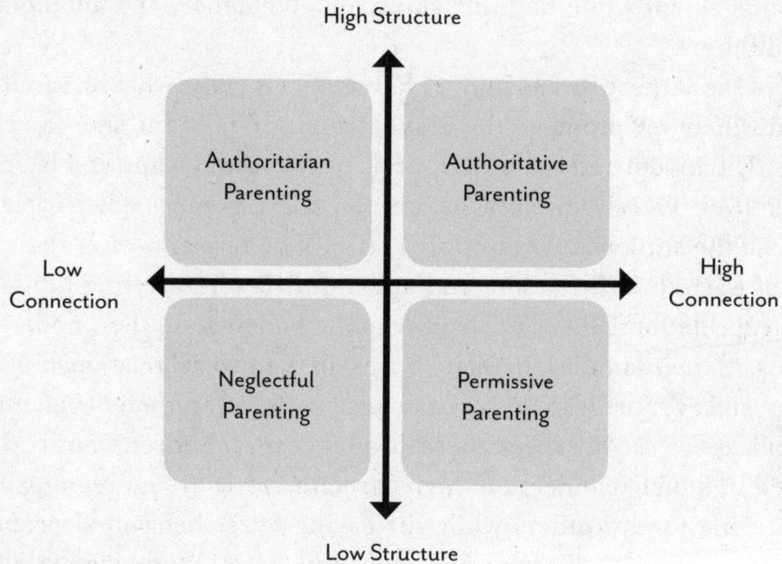

At the other extreme is a parent who's low on structure and high on connection, which puts his parenting style in the *permissive* camp. A permissive parent will regularly demonstrate warmth and emotional involvement, but he won't typically be consistent or firm when it comes to setting boundaries, placing limits, and expressing expectations for his kids' behavior. As a result, his parenting style will be characterized by leniency and even indulgence. This is Perspective #2, and in the diagram, it appears in the high-connection, low-structure quadrant.

Perspective #3 represents what happens when parents offer their children both high connection and high structure, resulting in what's called an *authoritative* parenting style. Here the parent will be both warm and nurturing while also setting clear boundaries and communicating high expectations. She will offer her kids consistent affection and affirmation for who they are, while simultaneously teaching them the meaning of "no" and helping them learn to regulate themselves, control their emotions and bodies, and make good decisions. In doing so, she'll be offering encouragement while building skills, independence, and autonomy in her children.

Looking at these three options, you can likely guess what research says about which one produces the best outcomes in both the short and long term. The model and the descriptions have evolved some and been adjusted over the last few decades, but the science comes down clearly in favor of the authoritative parenting style. When parents offer their kids lots of warmth, affirmation, and affection, all while setting limits and high expectations, their kids will reap the benefits—in their bodies and brains, in their families, in their classes, in their social relationships with peers, and eventually in their careers and as they start their own families.

And, as you might expect, there's evidence that children who are disciplined in a high-connection, high-structure style are more empathetic and caring toward others while displaying fewer behavioral problems and less aggression. They're even more advanced in terms of moral reasoning. You might find this somewhat counterintuitive and expect that the more rigid, authoritarian, my-way-or-the-highway parents would produce kids who at the very least were afraid to get out of line, ethically and morally. But authoritative parents—who offer high degrees of both connection and structure—encourage independent and critical thinking and collaborative communication, rather than simple obedience. As a result, their children are more likely to develop good decision-making abilities and get plenty of practice using their prefrontal cortex, the region of the brain in charge of things like self-control, decision-making, morality, empathy, critical thinking, resilience, and personal insight. Plus, since these parents emphasize the parent-child *relationship* so primarily, their kids are more likely to trust that they can go to them for advice as they become young adults and face difficult dilemmas without their parents becoming punitive or reactive. Studies show that children of more exclusively authoritarian or permissive parents are more apt to go to their peers for advice rather than their parents.

The fourth parenting style, by the way, describes parents who are low on both connection and structure. This is when you get what's called a neglectful parenting style, where the parent neither demands much of the child nor offers warmth and emotional responsiveness. Neglect is one of the most damaging realities for children and their developing brains, so if you or someone you know is neglecting a child (or abusing a child in some other way), it's important to get help and intervention right away.

One interesting aside regarding what the science says about parenting styles and discipline has to do with educational, ethnic, and socioeconomic differences. I won't go into a full discussion here, but there are studies showing that the positive outcomes associated with authoritative parenting don't always apply in the same way for children from lower socioeconomic groups, at least when it comes to academic success. Gwen Dewar, in her online article on the subject, surmises that kids who live in high-risk and dangerous environments may do better and get into less trouble if they're simply obedient, rather than thinking for themselves and questioning authority in ways that might be praised in a different setting. It's also true that some studies have shown that children of Chinese descent in Hong Kong and North America achieve better academic results when parented with an authoritarian style. But the author of one of these studies questions whether the term "authoritarian" is even correct in this case, since Chinese authoritarian parents typically develop more closeness with their children than their American counterparts do with theirs. Plus, even when an authoritarian parenting style produces better academic (or behavioral or athletic or other positive) outcomes, we often need to ask, "At what cost?"

So, as usual, complicating questions can arise when we're looking at research. But aside from certain exceptions, the science clearly argues that children will do much better in virtually all domains if their parents are emotionally attuned and responsive (high on connection), while also clearly communicating with their children about expectations and boundaries (high on structure).

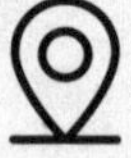

The Bottom Line

THE BOTTOM LINE here is a good bit longer than in other entries of the book, because I want to pull some practical ideas together on this important topic. (If you want a fuller treatment of what I discuss below, take a look at *No-Drama Discipline,* my book with Dan Siegel.) As with so many other aspects of parenting, this early period while your child is an infant is when you'll set the tone for how you think about and handle discipline, and what approach you want to take as you raise your child. You have the opportunity right now, during your child's first year, to lay the groundwork for an effective discipline approach that will pay dividends for years (and even generations!) to come.

Effective discipline is about a lot more than command, demand, and punish. The ultimate long-term goal of discipline is to raise a child who is *self-disciplined*. The way we do that is by reframing discipline moments as opportunities to teach and build skills. This requires that we begin to change how we think about our role as disciplinarians—we're actually teachers, not punishers. And if learning is the goal, so that our children handle themselves better in the future, then the combination of warmth *and* limit-setting is the best approach for making the brain most open to learning.

What does all of this mean, practically? Well, again, it's not the case that you don't have to worry about discipline until your baby is a toddler. And you will have plenty of teachable moments even in the first year, when baby bites at the breast (ouch!), throws food, reaches for an unsafe object, and more.

The goal is to commit yourself to being the kind of parent who consistently (not perfectly!) offers your child warmth and connection ("I can see you're upset and having a hard time; I will help you") while also teaching about boundaries and limit-setting ("You really want to touch that, but it's not safe"). If you can put those priorities into practice now and as your child moves into toddlerhood, your child will handle herself better not just during the good times but also when she faces difficult circumstances. She'll be better able to control her emotions and body, bounce back when things don't go her way, understand herself and her desires, and consider the feelings of others while responding with empathy. She'll feel safe when she knows what to expect, when limits and boundaries are explained to her and are predictable.

And it can begin with your infant, even before you're actively setting limits. As pediatric speech and language pathologist Hanna Bogen Novak puts it, "So much of the first year is about figuring out what it means to be a parent and keep your kid alive, while finding a rhythm as a new parent that you can maintain and grow into as your child grows. Those early routines, along with the verbal and behavioral modeling that come with them, create the social engagement with babies during the first year that *are* the beginnings of developing a positive discipline approach."

This isn't a how-to book, so I won't get too prescriptive here, but I'll stress a couple of key points regarding discipline. First of all, stay tuned in to your child. The more responsive and nurturing you are, the more proactive you can be in preventing discipline issues from coming up in the first place. For example, if you've told your child not to touch the breakable vase on the table, and she repeatedly wants to touch it, just put the vase away. I know someone will ask, "Don't they have to learn sometime?" Of course they do, and they will, but not at ten months old. Instead, set your baby up for success. You'll experience less oppositional behavior, both now and moving forward.

Also key is maintaining appropriate developmental expectations. A lot of discipline problems come when parents hold the expectation that a baby can do something—such as control themselves or make a good decision (or resist touching the vase on the table)—that in fact she can't do. Say you tell your eight-month-old not to throw food, and she immediately wings her green beans across the kitchen. If you believe your baby is capable of following directions and resisting certain temptations, then you're likely to see this as a discipline issue, or even a personal affront. It might even make you angry. But you don't want to punish your infant for being an infant. If you understand that an eight-month-old is likely experimenting with all kinds of skill building—gravity, physics, and motor skills are all being tested in the green-bean lab experiment right there in the high chair—and isn't developmentally prepared to follow directions or consider consequences in this way, then you'll be able to approach the situation with much more patience and understanding, all while offering structure and still setting limits.

And finally, we have to train ourselves as parents. The most important part of discipline the first year is building *our own* brain, orienting *ourselves* for how we want to handle defiance and the times when our kids don't respond to the limits we set. This first year is our basic training. It's boot camp for discipline so that we can (usually) be the kind of parent we want to be as they get older. That means practicing staying calm and learning how to handle our own reactivity in positive ways. We need to model remaining in control of ourselves even when emotions run high. When we blow up, yell, and lose control, our children don't feel secure and protected in that moment. They count on us to help them feel safe, and to demonstrate that even when they can't handle their big feelings and moods, we can. *They need to know that we'll help them when things get overwhelming, instead of contributing to their internal chaos.*

So monitor your own body and emotions, and when you feel frustration and anger building, pay attention to what's going on. Before you move into rage, take steps to calm yourself. Remove yourself from the situation for a minute if you have to, rather than doing something that might harm your baby.

You won't be perfect, but prioritize being warm and nurturing to the extent you can while you set limits ("I know you want to touch that, sweetie, but that's not safe for babies"). As Dan Siegel and I have stressed in the books we've written together, the best strategy is first to connect, then redirect. Do you notice the two dimensions there? Warmth first—where the child sees that you understand his desire—then boundaries. Connection, then structure. *Both* are important. Connect with your child first, then redirect him toward a more acceptable behavior. Let that become your habit as a parent and a disciplinarian, and you and your child, along with the relationship you two share, will be headed for success.

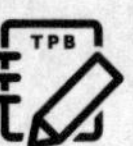

On a Personal Note

WHILE I WAS writing my doctoral dissertation on child rearing and studying attachment science and interpersonal neurobiology, I had small children. My discipline philosophy changed a lot over the years as I became more informed not only by the science—particularly about how the brain works and the role that safety and emotional regulation play in increasing a child's ability to learn—but also by trial and error. When I examined what I and so many others were doing in the name of discipline, I found myself repeatedly asking, "Can't we do this better?" Even as Baumrind's categorization proved very helpful, and I worked to be nurturing and respectful while still setting clear limits and expectations, I kept finding that many of my parental go-to techniques simply weren't that effective.

Along the way, I eventually had a "eureka" moment, when I got clear on the fact that discipline really is about teaching. And *so many* of our disciplinary approaches aren't only ineffective; they're actually counterproductive! I saw that many of my discipline techniques didn't make a lot of sense because they didn't do anything to help my children learn or build skills or do things differently the next time. Far too often, my responses to their behavior actually distracted them from receiving the lessons I wanted them to absorb.

I remember the time I sent my three-year-old to time-out, and he refused to stay there. I ended up chasing him around the house, and when I caught him, I restrained him (gently) to enforce my authority; he resisted, of course. As the battle escalated, we both ended up so upset that neither of us even remembered what the original infraction was in the first place. I wasn't gaining compliance, and he wasn't building skills for the future. No teaching whatsoever was taking place.

At that moment, I saw it. My well-intentioned belief that I needed to punish my son so that he would be a functioning human later in life had eclipsed the goal of teaching him. It was counterproductive to what I was trying to help him learn.

From that moment, I've worked to focus on what discipline is actually about—yes, gaining cooperation, but also building skills for both now and the future. As a result, my discipline has become more effective in the short term, and more focused on teaching skills and helping my kids make better decisions overall in the long term. Just as our children's brains develop and get stronger from practice and experiences, ours do too, and the more we practice calm, responsive limit-setting and set empathetic boundaries, the easier and more automatic doing so can become.

Dream Feeding

"Dream feeding" describes the practice of strategically timing feedings to maximize the sleep of both baby and caregiver. The idea is to get a sleeping baby to feed without actually waking up. Some people use the phrase to refer to the idea of holding a baby while she's still sleeping and offering the breast or bottle. Others describe a dream feed as the act of deliberately waking a sleeping infant to feed just before the parent goes to bed, thus allowing the baby to sleep longer so the parent can as well. Is this a valid strategy?

Competing Opinions

Perspective #1: Dream feeding can help train your infant to sleep through the night. Correctly done, it won't disrupt a baby's sleep rhythm, and it can allow a mom or dad to get more shut-eye.

Perspective #2: Dream feeding doesn't work for all infants and can, in fact, make it harder for babies to get back to sleep. Plus, it may be difficult to rouse deeply sleeping babies enough to feed at all. And even if you find it helpful, how do you know when your baby can make it through the night without dream feeding? Most important, do you really want to wake a sleeping baby? Ever?

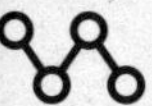

What the Science Says

WHILE THERE IS research looking at methods of sleep training in young infants, none has looked only at dream feeding. Some researchers have examined the practice as part of an overall sleep protocol, but even when that protocol leads to better sleep outcomes, it's not clear how much credit to give dream feeding, when the study is also exploring, for example, the use of swaddling, or white noise, or pacifiers, or other recommendations.

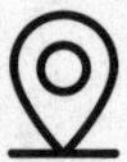

The Bottom Line

IN THE ABSENCE of any research on the effects of dream feeding as an isolated variable, you're left to decide without the guidance of scientific experts. The logic behind the practice does make sense, though, assuming your baby is otherwise healthy. If you can help him "tank up" just before you get into bed, it might give you a better chance of taking advantage of the deep, restorative non–rapid eye movement (NREM) sleep of the early sleep cycles of the night. Especially if you combine it with other sleep-encouraging practices, it might be one more strategy that helps buy you an extra few hours of rest. If it doesn't help, or if you determine that you're actually interfering with your baby's sleep, then you can simply end the practice and try something else.

Ear Piercing

Piercing has been around for centuries, often as an important practice with religious, cultural, and family significance. But is it safe to pierce your baby's ears?

Competing Opinions

Perspective #1: As long as you're careful with the procedure and conscientious about caring for the wound afterward, there's no reason not to participate in this traditional practice.

Perspective #2: For one thing, ear piercing causes babies pain. Sometimes pain is necessary, as when we decide to give them certain shots. But at least then it's for a necessary, medical reason. In the case of piercing, the parent has made the decision for the child, without the baby having a vote, to cause pain for cosmetic reasons. On top of everything, it can lead to medical complications.

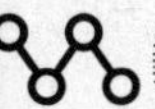

What the Science Says

THERE'S NOT MUCH research to guide us in this question. Studies have been performed regarding ear piercing and other "body modifications" in general. A number have focused specifically on children and adolescents. But when it comes to infants, we don't have much data to go on aside from guidelines from various authorities and organizations.

What we do know is that, broadly speaking, piercings can lead to complications when proper precautions aren't taken. The list is long and includes pain, allergic reactions, undesired cosmetic effects, and even serious infections such as hepatitis and HIV. Babies aren't immune to these negative outcomes, and obviously their vulnerability should lead parents to be even more cautious when considering these realities. Another concern is the ingestion of the earring if an infant finds it.

Still, despite these risks, infant ear piercing can be safe as long as the procedure is performed correctly and the wound is well cared for. The most specific set of recommendations we receive from a body of authorities comes from the AAP, which affirms that ears may be pierced "at any age." In a statement regarding infection and ear piercing, the group emphasizes the importance of the process and the environment of the procedure itself: "If the piercing is performed carefully and cared for conscientiously, there is little risk, no matter what the age of the child. However, as a general guideline, postpone the piercing until your child is mature enough to take care of the pierced site herself."

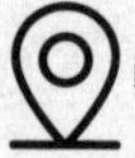

The Bottom Line

IF YOUR FAMILY'S or culture's tradition is to pierce an infant's ears, then there's really no scientific reason not to do so. Just keep in mind the importance of having the procedure completed in a sterile environment by a qualified person who can guide you in post-procedure care. I agree with the AAP, which encourages having a doctor, nurse, or experienced technician perform the procedure. It's also a good idea to wait until after the second round of vaccinations and your pediatrician has signed off on your baby's overall health.

Elimination Communication

A form of toilet training known as "elimination communication" (EC) or "infant toilet training" has become an alternative approach to traditional potty training for some in the United States. The idea is for the parent and baby to establish communication about elimination, meaning that the parent gets used to understanding the infant's natural timing and recognizing cues that the baby is about to pee or poop. The parent can then quickly put the baby on the toilet or potty chair, holding the child in place if he is too young to sit up by himself. As a result, diapers are much less necessary.

But is it practical? And does it really potty-train your baby?

Competing Opinions

Perspective #1: Some form of EC is the norm throughout parts of Asia, Africa, and Latin America. And with an estimated 27.4 billion disposable diapers used every year in the United States, the idea of toilet training your infant more naturally, without depending on disposable or cloth diapers, makes a lot of sense ecologically and financially.

EC eliminates a reliance on disposable or cloth diapers to the benefit of the environment and your wallet. It also encourages more complete emptying of the bladder, helping prevent urinary tract infections, irritation of the skin, and skin infections like MRSA (methicillin-resistant *Staphylococcus aureus*). Yes, there will be some messes, but along the way EC will teach kids to recognize their own bodily signals; they won't learn to ignore them simply because they have the security of wearing diapers.

Perspective #2: Being more in tune with your infant is of course a good thing, but are the potential benefits of EC worth putting up with what's required to "potty-train" an infant? The messiness alone will give some parents pause. But beyond that, EC is time-consuming work and requires constant close supervision and consistency by all caregivers for a long period. Most families can't devote that kind of time. Plus, it's not even toilet training, because infants are not developmentally ready for this type of body-awareness and decision-making. It's good to help kids understand their bodily signals, but at some point they'll still have to learn about walking to the toilet, wiping, dealing with clothes, and so on.

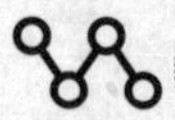

What the Science Says

THERE'S ALMOST NO research on this particular subject. One study that looked at EC did find that babies indeed give signs of needing to eliminate and concluded that children whose parents used the strategy beginning in the first six months were trained by seventeen months on average. The study also found no adverse results from working with babies this young.

As for health benefits, practicing EC would mean keeping your baby out of soiled diapers, as well as promoting the complete emptying of the bladder, both of which could reduce the risk of urinary tract infections and MRSA.

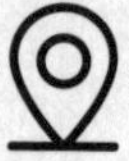

The Bottom Line

EC DOESN'T SEEM to affect babies in any adverse way. Likewise, there's no evidence that it somehow benefits children or their relationship with their parents. So your decision will depend on whether you have the patience, time, and inclination to do it.

Also, it's important to keep in mind that beginning EC with your baby in the first few months of life isn't going to lead to having a potty-trained child anytime soon. Toilet independence requires a level of developmental maturity that simply doesn't appear until your child can crawl or walk

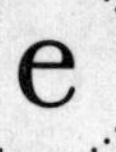

to a designated place, twelve to eighteen months at the earliest. It's not until that age that kids can control their bowels and bladder, and most can't do it until twenty-four to thirty months.

Ultimately, while many parents throughout the world practice some form of elimination communication, it may not be a practical or particularly convenient method for most parents. EC may help prevent certain infections and irritations, and it offers some financial and ecological benefits, but it requires a consistent commitment that may prove more burdensome than beneficial for many families.

Whatever you decide, and however you decide to toilet-train, first spend some time thinking about how you want to handle the inevitable frustration you'll feel during your child's stops and starts throughout the process. If you use pressure in an attempt at quick success, when your child may not be developmentally ready for a good while, that won't be good for either of you, or for your relationship. Even very young children pick up on parental negative emotions such as frustration, and it could turn the whole ordeal into a negative experience. The brain makes associations between related events, so if using the bathroom is linked in the child's mind to Mommy being mad or Daddy turning it into a big control thing, then your child may develop a negative association with using the bathroom or toilet, meaning you'll likely have an even longer battle on your hands.

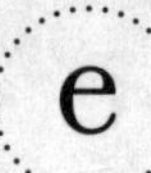

Extended Breastfeeding

Breastfeeding clearly offers numerous benefits, but how long should it last? Nursing beyond a baby's first birthday is considered extended breastfeeding in the United States and in many other Western cultures. Worldwide, however, babies are weaned on average between the ages of two and four years. Is this just a matter of personal preference?

Competing Opinions

Perspective #1: If both baby and mother feel good about it, and it works for them, then why not keep breastfeeding? Assuming you follow guidelines about supplementing with complementary foods along the way, breastfeeding longer than twelve months provides health and relational benefits for both mother and infant. More time breastfeeding continues to boost a child's immunities and can lower the mother's risk of certain illnesses. It also can further strengthen the parent-child bond and provide a powerful tool for soothing an upset toddler.

Perspective #2: It's not that extended breastfeeding is somehow *bad;* it's just that it can produce unwanted consequences. One is obviously the reactions of others that come when a larger child is still breastfeeding in public. Also, it can make weaning more difficult when the time comes. Older kids may even demand to be breastfed in ways and in places that some others consider inappropriate.

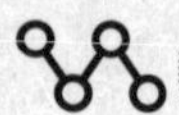

What the Science Says

WHEREAS RESEARCH AND health authorities are clear about the many health benefits associated with breastfeeding—including bolstered immunity for the child, and for the mother a reduced risk of breast and ovarian can-

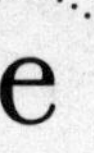

cers, heart disease, high blood pressure, type 2 diabetes, and rheumatoid arthritis—extended breastfeeding hasn't been studied to nearly the same extent. Still, various studies have found that breast milk provides important protein, fat, and vitamins well beyond the first year of life. For the purposes of our discussion here, I'll define extended breastfeeding as breastfeeding between one and three years of age.

In addition to the health benefits, breastfeeding also helps with mother-child bonding. A longitudinal study published in 2017 found that women who breastfeed their children longer (up to age three) exhibit more "maternal sensitivity" well past the infant and toddler years, with mothers showing more sensitivity even up until the child reaches age eleven. The same study found that this extended nursing correlates with secure attachment, or a strong parent-child bond with lifelong benefits, including independence in the child.

One potential negative associated with extended breastfeeding involves dental issues. There has been some dispute in the research, but it does appear that prolonged breastfeeding increases the risk of early childhood caries (decay or crumbling of a tooth or bone). The authors of one study take the step of recommending that preventative measures be established for care of teeth—checkups, cleaning, and other maintenance—as early as possible, "because breastfeeding is beneficial for children's health."

Leading health organizations continue to endorse extended breastfeeding, despite the dental concerns. The AAP recommends breastfeeding for one year or longer as mutually desired by the mother and baby, and the World Health Organization and UNICEF recommend that breastfeeding continue until age two or longer, suggesting that it be frequent and on-demand.

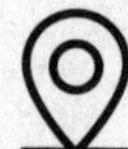

The Bottom Line

IN 1990, THE psychiatrist and former U.S. surgeon general Antonia Novello declared, "It's the lucky baby . . . who continues to nurse until he's two." Large groups of pediatricians and researchers who study the issue, bolstered by the still-limited science available, agree with Novell's often-referenced quote. If you can nurse your baby for an extended time, you'll be offering him a number of potential advantages.

That being said, *any* number of months of breastfeeding provides benefits, so if you nurse for only a few months or through the end of the first year, you're already giving your baby a lot of advantages. Extended breastfeeding is not for everyone. Some mothers aren't able to nurse that long, because of their bodies, their schedules, or some other dynamic. And some children will wean themselves earlier than others, even before a mother is ready to stop. If you're not able to nurse into your child's second or third year, there's no reason to despair—you can celebrate what you've already done. You can still provide your infant with the necessary nutrition, and you two will have more than enough opportunities to connect with each other and build a strong bond.

If you have the opportunity and the inclination, though, continue nursing as your infant becomes a toddler. Be sure to supplement his nutrition by getting him plenty of fruits, vegetables, and grains, as well as foods or supplements that provide the necessary amounts of iron and vitamin D. And if you worry about others judging you for breastfeeding as your baby gets older, there are plenty of ways to establish routines that help your toddler understand about privacy and about your boundaries regarding breastfeeding on demand.

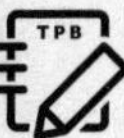

On a Personal Note

BEFORE I HAD babies, I never expected to nurse past age one, but for each of them, when they reached their first birthday, I changed my mind. They were still so little, and I ended up nursing longer and longer with each of my three. I didn't end up missing it after those years were over, because I felt like I had been all in. At the same time, I didn't regret one day of doing it as long as I did. Those infant and toddler nursing years were really sweet, special times with each of my kids for that particular season of life, and while I definitely felt limited at times because I was breastfeeding, those years were gone in what seemed like no time at all.

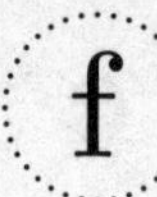

First Bath

Should you bathe your baby as soon as she's born? Or delay her first bath for a day or two?

Competing Opinions

Perspective #1: As a general rule, it's good to be clean. Bathing newborns shortly after birth reduces the risk of infection by limiting the presence of germs. Parents can feel good about protecting their child and being conscientious about health from the very beginning. Plus, if there's bacteria in the environment, or if the mother has some sort of transmitted illness—if she's HIV positive or has hepatitis or a staph infection, for example—then bathing her infant will protect the baby and anyone who comes into contact with the newborn.

Perspective #2: Babies aren't born dirty, and they don't come out of the womb needing an immediate bath. The fluids covering the body are important and should be allowed to do their work, providing health benefits. In addition, waiting can give the baby time to adjust to her new surroundings without introducing another potentially unpleasant experience.

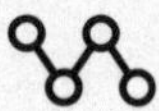

What the Science Says

SINCE THE EARLY 1900S, amid concerns about germs, the standard practice has been for nurses to bathe hospital-born babies within hours of birth. However, recent research suggests that delaying the first bath may be more beneficial.

The World Health Organization recommends delaying the first bath for at least twenty-four hours—or at least six hours if certain cultural factors mandate an earlier cleansing. The AAP agrees. Delaying the first bath increases the rates of effective breastfeeding, since it can preserve the amniotic-fluid smell on the baby, which is comparable to the smell of the breast. What's more, if you avoid an immediate bath, you preserve the waxy coating, called vernix caseosa, on your newborn's skin. This coating provides a natural moisturizer and cleanser that protects against infection and helps the skin adapt to the new environment after birth.

Newborn babies aren't yet adept at regulating their body temperature. They have thin skin and are less capable of generating heat, leaving them vulnerable if they get too cold before, during, or after the bath. Bathing, therefore, can create a stressful experience. It can also hinder the ideal immediate postpartum experience, in which mother-infant skin-to-skin bonding and breastfeeding time are maximized, and the newborn's separation from the mother is minimized.

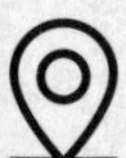

The Bottom Line

BABIES ARE NOT born contaminated and in fact have natural protection against becoming so. More and more hospitals and midwives are delaying bathing newborns, primarily to allow for more immediate bonding time between mother and infant. If you're nervous about postponing the first bath, you can wipe around the neck and diaper area with a wet cloth. But ideally, wait several hours, if not a day or two, to bathe a healthy newborn. (For more details, see "Bathing.")

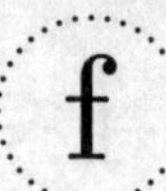

Food Allergens and Early Exposure

Is it best to expose babies to potentially allergenic foods early on? Or to avoid them until a much later time?

Competing Opinions

Perspective #1: Exposing infants to potentially allergenic foods at an early age (four to six months) may help build tolerance and prevent future allergies, even for infants with a family history of reactions to certain foods.

Perspective #2: Delaying the introduction of potentially allergenic foods helps to prevent allergies in the long term. This is particularly advisable for high-risk infants with a family history of food allergies.

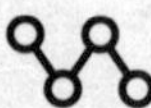

What the Science Says

THE EVIDENCE IS becoming increasingly clear that introducing potentially allergenic foods (such as peanuts, fish, and eggs) early—sometime after four to six months—can be helpful in preventing food allergies, and that delaying such introductions might actually lead to an increase in those allergies. A 2008 study found that children who began eating peanuts before one year of age displayed fewer peanut allergies later than children who were not exposed at an early age. A 2010 analysis found that infants introduced to eggs between four and six months had a lower rate of egg allergies than infants introduced to them at twelve months. Other studies have drawn similar conclusions. In 2019, a meta-analysis observed that introducing eggs at around four to six months and peanuts anywhere from four to eleven months reduced the risk associated with egg and peanut allergies.

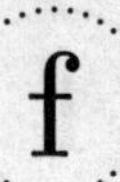

As a result of findings such as these, leading health organizations have declared that there is no allergy-related reason to delay introducing solid foods after six months of age. The American Academy of Pediatrics has stated more than once that while parents should wait until a child is four to six months of age to introduce solid foods, there is no compelling allergy-related evidence to delay food introduction beyond this period. In 2013 the Canadian Paediatric Society and the Canadian Society of Allergy and Clinical Immunology agreed, declaring that there's no benefit to delaying the introduction of potentially allergenic foods (milk, eggs, peanuts, and fish) beyond six months. The WHO, the European Society for Pediatric Gastroenterology, Hepatology and Nutrition, and the Asia Pacific Association of Pediatric Allergy, Respirology and Immunology have all followed suit in one way or another.

There are non-allergy-related exceptions. For example, cow's milk is often discouraged for a child's first year, simply because it's hard for a baby's system to handle the high levels of nutrients in cow's (or goat's or soy) milk. Avoid honey as well, not because it causes allergies but because it's been associated with infant botulism. Both the U.S. Food and Drug Administration and the Centers for Disease Control and Prevention advise against giving babies honey before the age of one; this includes pacifiers dipped in honey.

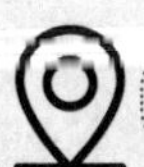

The Bottom Line

IN THE PAST, parents were routinely advised to delay the introduction of certain foods that were considered allergenic, particularly peanuts, milk, and eggs. More recent research suggests that exposure to these foods should not be avoided. Rather, their early introduction may help to create a tolerance for them. (Obviously, parents should always be careful to consider any choking hazard associated with certain solid foods, such as peanuts, and watch for any allergic reactions just in case.)

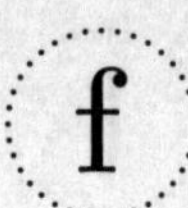

THE BOTTOM LINE FOR BABY

As for the exact timing of introducing different foods, you should consult with your pediatrician. But as a general rule of thumb, it's a good idea to begin introducing potentially allergenic foods once your baby is four to six months old. If you or your partner has allergies or if they run in your families, it's even more important to discuss food introduction with your trusted pediatrician.

Germs

In 1989, the British epidemiologist David Strachan introduced what came to be called the "hygiene hypothesis" to explain an increase in hay fever during the twentieth century. He pointed to the decreasing size of the family and higher standards of cleanliness as factors that had, ironically, led to higher rates of illness. The basic idea was that as kids were exposed to less dirt and fewer microorganisms overall, their immune systems weren't responding by developing and becoming stronger, but instead were becoming weaker, resulting in more sickness, especially allergies. Evidently, according to Strachan, modern society was becoming too sanitized for its own good!

Many parents, whether they know of Strachan or not, have heard the basic idea of the hygiene hypothesis and rightly wonder, how clean is too clean? Is it better to expose an infant to germs, or is conscientious protection a safer alternative?

Competing Opinions

Perspective #1: Exposing an infant to common household germs and dirt will help them develop a strong immune system. Oversanitizing an environment will cause a baby's immune system to remain immature or become hypersensitized, rather than developing strength and resilience.

Perspective #2: Newborns have weak immune systems, so it's only common sense that vigilant care should be taken to protect them from exposure to germs. Parents should frequently use soap, hand sanitizers, and other antibacterial products. They should also keep household surfaces free of germs and make sure anyone who touches their newborn washes their hands first.

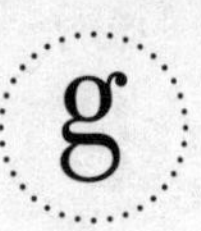

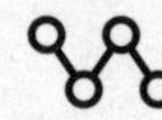

What the Science Says

AS ONE RESEARCHER puts it, "It is becoming clear that a symbiotic relationship exists between bacteria and our immune system," and that children benefit from being exposed to certain microbes. Of course parents need to protect their babies from infections carried by others and be smart about what they expose them to, especially in public places like malls, hospitals, and airplanes. But it definitely appears to be the case that children's health can also suffer when we become overprotective in terms of germs and cleanliness.

One of the best-known recent studies to support this growing awareness compared children from contemporary Amish communities, where kids grow up following traditional farming practices on single-family farms (with the expected high level of microbes) with those of Hutterite communities, which typically have large, industrialized farms with more antiseptic environments. Researchers found that the Amish kids were much less likely to develop asthma and allergic sensitization than the Hutterite kids. This was found despite the fact that the two groups share similar genetic makeups.

Other findings support the hygiene hypothesis, demonstrating, for example, that risk for eczema goes down when a parent tends to suck a dropped pacifier clean rather than washing it. Likewise, as gross as it may seem, exposing newborns to germs, pet and rodent dander, and roach allergens can lower the risk of developing asthma and allergies. Even thumb sucking and nail biting are correlated with a decreased risk of asthma and hay fever.

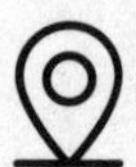

The Bottom Line

WHILE HUMAN BABIES are born with natural protections against many germs, it would be irresponsible to deliberately expose a newborn, whose immune system is still developing, to someone who is ill. And especially until your child has been vaccinated, try to steer clear of sick children who haven't had their shots, as some childhood illnesses can be dangerous for young babies. If a baby less than two months old develops a fever, she will need to be seen by a doctor and may need to be tested because young infants cannot contain their infections as well as older children and adults. So having hand sanitizer and masks available for visitors who are ill and allowing other children to kiss only the top of your baby's head are wise measures during the first two months.

That said, oversanitizing an infant's environment is not only unnecessary but likely to deprive the child of health benefits and resilience down the road. Let your baby get into some messes, and do your best to enjoy those typically cringeworthy moments—like the times your dog licks the applesauce off your child's face—knowing that those experiences are fortifying your baby's immune system.

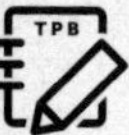

On a Personal Note

I HEARD A funny take on this issue as it relates to birth order. If your firstborn eats dirt, you call the pediatrician. If your second eats dirt, you rinse their mouth and give them a nutritious snack. If your third eats dirt, you shrug and say, "Well, now I don't have to make lunch." It's true that we typically become more comfortable and less fear-driven the longer we parent. We learn that many of the things we worried about the first time around aren't huge deals.

Introducing Solid Foods

When your baby is about six months old she will probably be ready for solid foods. You want to wait until she can stay vertical—holding her head steady and sitting upright without support—so that she can swallow well and avoid choking.

But what foods do you introduce first? Do you start with easy-to-digest foods, such as rice cereal? And do you worry about foods that are more likely to trigger an allergic reaction?

Competing Opinions

Perspective #1: Solid foods should be offered in an order that's gentler on an infant's digestive system, beginning with cereals, then fruits, vegetables, and finally the harder-to-digest proteins. Make sure, too, to avoid or at least delay the introduction of common allergens, like wheat, eggs, fish, and peanut and milk products.

Perspective #2: When your baby is ready for solid foods, you can introduce a variety of foods without stressing her digestive system. There's no hard-and-fast rule that you need to introduce cereals first, or that you need to worry about allergens.

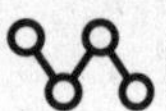

What the Science Says

IN THE PAST, parents were counseled to introduce their infants first to an easy-to-digest and non-allergenic diet, then work their way toward other, "complementary" solid foods. More recently, though, research studies and health organizations are suggesting that parents not worry about the order in which solid foods are introduced. Instead, the AAP says that there's no medical evidence that supports beginning with, say, single-grain cereals. Obviously, you should be mindful of choking hazards, and if there's a history of allergy in your family, you should be especially careful and communicate with your pediatrician. But generally speaking, babies can eat a variety of foods—infant cereals, fruits and vegetables, grains, proteins, and yogurts and cheeses—and the order does not matter.

Some people will tell you that you should begin with vegetables before fruits because once you introduce the sweeter fruits there will be no going back to less exciting veggies. But this may be an old wives' tale; there's no evidence that babies who have fruits first will end up disliking vegetables. It also doesn't appear that the order in which you choose to introduce foods will affect whether your baby has a strong desire for sweets. Babies, like all of us, are typically born with that preference.

When it comes to the best time to introduce solid foods, after six months you can do so with certainty. Earlier than that and there's a bit of scientific murkiness. For example, one study warns against beginning too early, finding that introducing solids before four months of age is associated with childhood obesity, but other studies are finding definite benefits (such as reduced allergy risk and greater willingness to try new foods) to introducing certain solids as early as four months. At this point the research isn't clear on this question, so the majority of experts still recommend exclusive nursing for the first six months of a child's life. Still, the AAP notes that "when infants double their birth weight (typically at about 4 months of age) and weigh about 13 pounds or more, they may be ready for solid foods."

As for the question of potentially allergenic foods after six months, the short answer is that you don't have to worry about it. I've discussed the question more fully in the entry "Food Allergens and Early Exposure," but suffice it to say that you can, and probably should, be introducing your baby to foods that parents used to shy away from, like peanuts, fish, and eggs. Doing so seems to actually prevent those food allergies.

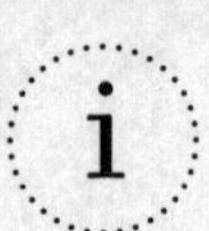

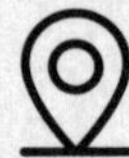

The Bottom Line

IF YOUR BABY can sit up and bring objects to her mouth, she's likely ready to have her diet expanded to include solid foods. Assuming you're avoiding choking hazards and paying attention to family patterns related to allergies, you can relax and feel free to offer her a variety of foods from different food groups.

Keep in mind that when introducing your baby to solid foods, you're laying the groundwork for how she feels about eating and mealtime. You're introducing her to her relationship with food and laying tracks of association in her brain. If mealtimes with your baby are full of parental frustration, anger, or punitiveness (I recently heard about a parent flicking the cheek of an infant if the child drops food), your child may associate eating or mealtimes with something that's unpleasant to be avoided. If you want to create in your infant healthy associations with food and eating with the family, then make sure you're creating a positive environment.

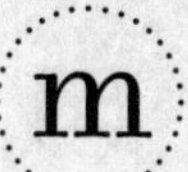

Marijuana and Breastfeeding

As marijuana makes gains in terms of legalization and acceptance of its medical benefits, have we reached a point where breastfeeding mothers can use it in good conscience?

Competing Opinions

Perspective #1: Marijuana can be safely consumed in limited quantities by lactating mothers, with minimal effects on the infant.

Perspective #2: Marijuana is dangerous not only because it gets transferred to the breast milk but also because of the dangers of exposing the baby to secondhand smoke. It's just too risky.

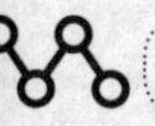

What the Science Says

IT HAS NOT yet been ascertained whether exposure through breast milk to tetrahydrocannabinol (THC), the main psychoactive compound in marijuana, produces long-term harm in infants, and some of the evidence available is limited and even conflicting. Research has shown, though, that THC can be absorbed and metabolized by babies, and data suggests at least the potential for harm, including impaired brain development and risks associated with secondhand smoke, which correlates with a risk of sudden infant death syndrome (SIDS).

A 2018 review of recent systematic reviews and meta-analyses ultimately concludes with the advice to doctors that they advise women "to refrain from using marijuana during pregnancy and lactation." Most national health organizations—the American Academy of Pediatrics, the American College of Obstetricians and Gynecologists, the Academy of

Breastfeeding Medicine, and others—agree, recommending at least extreme caution, if not complete abstinence, regarding cannabis use during lactation.

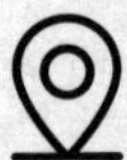

The Bottom Line

LIMITED STUDIES SUGGEST that exposing your infant to THC through breast milk directly or through secondhand smoke from marijuana could interfere with normal brain development. More research is taking place at the moment, and we'll have additional data in a few years. But at the moment, based on what we know, the bottom line is clear: the healthy development of your baby is too important to risk an exposure to the potential repercussions associated with marijuana use, whether you smoke it or ingest it in some other way.

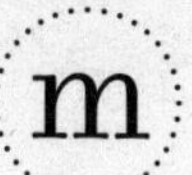

Massage

Baby massage is used all over the world, and has been for centuries. It's now becoming a more prevalent practice in the United States, with promises of not only better sleep, respiration, elimination, and growth but also less colic and stress for the baby. Should you be massaging your baby?

Competing Opinions

Perspective #1: Baby massage is a great way to bond with your baby, and it offers a multitude of benefits. It's a free, simple, and fun way to encourage your child's optimal development.

Perspective #2: The science isn't clear that baby massage is helpful or important, and it can even be harmful. A baby's skin is delicate, and if you're not gentle enough, or if you use an oil that can break down the skin's protective barriers, you could do damage.

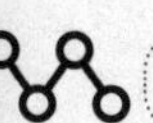

What the Science Says

THERE'S NO DOUBT, according to the research literature, that touch is powerful and necessary for a baby's development. Skin-to-skin contact with infants has been shown to promote social development, encourage brain growth, lower stress levels, and increase relational trust. It can also improve breastfeeding and increase a newborn's overall contentment.

As for research specifically devoted to baby massage, the science isn't quite as clear and specific. Numerous studies point to various benefits, but many of these are methodologically limited. Still, the research on the skin-to-skin benefits alone is powerful, not to mention the increased parent-child bonding that accompanies baby massage. And the research continues to evolve and support claims about the positive effects of infant massage. For newborns in the neonatal intensive care unit (NICU), for instance, massage appears to help reduce the length of stay, reduce pain, and improve weight gain. It also can improve the experience of parents of babies in NICU, resulting in less stress, anxiety, and depression. In fact, a 2017 study found that the experience of massaging a baby improves a parent's overall attitude regarding childbearing and produces greater satisfaction and pleasure in parenting.

On the question of whether to use oils, and which ones are acceptable, the science is often conflicting. But most experts advise that you choose an unscented, edible cold-pressed fruit, nut, seed, or vegetable oil. A baby's skin is delicate and should be vigorously protected. (See the entry "Sunscreen.")

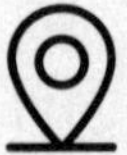

The Bottom Line

GIVEN THAT INFANT massage offers certain benefits—chief among them that it promotes parent-child bonding—and that it doesn't come with any proven drawbacks, there's really no reason not to massage your infant. One caveat is that if your child has a skin condition or other medical issue, you should be sure to check with your pediatrician to be aware of any risks related to your child's particular situation. Educate yourself about some infant massage basics you might not be aware of. For example, you want to massage a baby's belly in a clockwise direction around the navel, since the colon starts on the right side and if you massage in a counterclockwise direction, the baby could experience some constipation. Also, be sure to read about the pros and cons of using certain oils, and avoid talcum and baby powders. (See the entry "Baby Powder.") Finally, be gentle, and, as always, follow your baby's cues, watching for signs that she's not in the mood or has had enough for one session.

And watch for signs that you yourself might need a massage. It's a great way to promote your own relaxation and care.

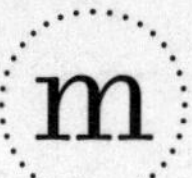

Medications and Breastfeeding

Should mothers avoid medications when breastfeeding? How concerned should you be if you need to take something when you're sick?

Competing Opinions

Perspective #1: If you get sick, it's best to either wean your baby or make it through the illness without taking medication. Virtually any drug you take will make its way to your breast milk, and some medications can concentrate especially strongly. Why take chances?

Perspective #2: Of course you should be smart about which drugs you take and for how long, but the benefits of taking a medication for a health condition generally outweigh the risk to your nursing baby.

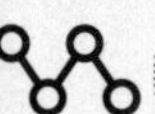

What the Science Says

THE CDC SUMMARIZES the answer to the question clearly and simply: "Although many medications do pass into breast milk, most have little or no effect on milk supply or on infant well-being." Multiple studies and reports support this opinion, including an American Academy of Pediatrics policy statement on which the CDC position is based. In the case of depression specifically, some have argued that the benefits of breastfeeding outweigh the risks that might be associated with antidepressants, but many factors come into play with that decision.

As you might expect, therefore, all experts point out the importance of carefully considering risks and benefits of any drug before taking it, and doing so under the care of a physician. Extra caution should be taken with newborns and preterm babies. The risk of any type of contamination is lower once infants reach six months, when their bodies have developed fully enough to efficiently process whatever medicine might make it into their bloodstream from your milk supply.

Some medicines and classes of drugs—certain pain medications (such as codeine), specific antidepressants, and particular medications to address addiction—should be avoided, as should drugs of abuse. It's also the case that some medicines can affect milk production. Ibuprofen and acetaminophen are typically good ways to treat pain, but as always, check with your doctor and/or pharmacist before taking one of these medicines while breastfeeding. And in case you're wondering about herbal remedies, the jury is still out for the most part; studies show that some may actually be harmful, but for most we simply don't have the research yet.

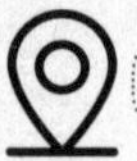

The Bottom Line

IT'S TRUE THAT medication that enters your bloodstream will transfer to your milk to some degree. And yes, certain drugs can have negative effects on a nursing child. Check with your pediatrician or a pharmacist before you take medication, but it's unlikely that you need to stop breastfeeding your infant if you get sick. When you can, you probably want to avoid long-acting forms of medications, which will remain in your body longer, and you should keep an eye out for any unusual behavior or symptoms in your child. (For the latest information about specific medications and how they affect lactating mothers and their children, see the NIH LactMed Drugs and Lactation online database.) But in the end, as long as you're being smart, doing your homework, and consulting with your doctor or your child's pediatrician, you should be able to get the relief and healing you need and protect your baby at the same time.

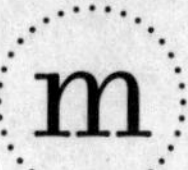

Music

You've heard about the Mozart effect: babies become smarter when their parents expose them to music, classical or otherwise. Is there any truth to the claim?

Competing Opinions

Perspective #1: Research shows that music improves kids' intelligence by introducing them to rhythms, rhymes, and patterns. It enhances brain development and helps them learn, and can even improve their social interactions.

Perspective #2: The claim that music makes a baby smarter is based on old research that showed very minor improvement in college students' IQ scores when they listened to classical music before taking a test. People took the conclusions of that study and expanded them to make claims about children and babies that aren't based in science. There's nothing wrong with playing music for your infant, but don't expect it to lead to a Nobel Prize someday.

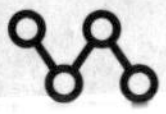

What the Science Says

WHILE RESEARCH IS still emerging, it appears more and more certain that exposing a baby to music offers lots of advantages. Neuroscientists have found actual changes in the brain—infants' auditory and prefrontal cortexes look different after the babies listen to music. It appears that these changes produce numerous health- and brain-related benefits.

For preterm infants specifically, the literature supports the use of music in helping babies sleep better, gain weight, and recover from painful procedures. One study published by the AAP showed that playing lullabies and simulating the whooshing sounds heard in the womb can offer numerous benefits for preterm babies, including improvements in bonding, feeding behaviors, and sucking patterns, as well as prolonged periods of quiet alertness. This study also found that singing lullabies live resulted in enhanced relational bonding and decreased stress for parents.

In addition, researchers have found that various kinds of music can help babies process speech more effectively and improve their understanding of rhythm in both speech and melody. Another study showed that when babies are exposed to interactive music classes, they smile more and communicate better, while also developing more sophisticated brain responses when exposed to other music. Further research points to positive traits resulting from kids listening to music as they grow into toddlerhood and the school years, including being more helpful, sharing, cooperative, empathetic, and trusting.

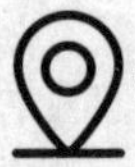

The Bottom Line

PLAY THOSE TUNES for your baby, and if you like to sing, then sing to your little one as well. Be sure to protect her delicate ears when it comes to volume (see the entry "Silence vs. Noise in the House"), but rest assured that music can offer her many advantages. Research doesn't set an exact amount of time for listening, and it doesn't prioritize genres. It just says that music produces these good results. So at home, in the car, and during your daily activities, expose your child to music.

Use it for yourself as well. In therapy sessions, I've sometimes "prescribed" music to families I'm working with, to transform the morning routine into a less stressful and more playful one. I've often heard back from parents that they find music a great tool that helps them be more patient and less reactive.

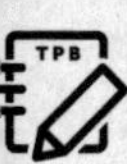

On a Personal Note

OUR HOUSE IS a musical one, and it always has been. The research showing how powerful music is in stimulating a child's brain is one reason my husband and I have played a lot of music for our kids through the years. But the main reason is that we all enjoy it so much.

When our oldest was a toddler, my husband got tired of the typical children's music. Unable to tolerate one more chorus of "Wheels on the Bus," he created a playlist with adult songs our young son liked and responded to but that we could enjoy as well: the Beatles, Aretha Franklin, Johnny Cash, Foo Fighters, and on and on. He made more and more playlists through the years, and these have been the sound track of our boys' childhoods. The musicians and genres evolved as the boys grew up, but they heard music all the time: at breakfast, while doing their chores, while playing, in the van on the way to a game.

We worked hard to screen our kids from inappropriate language and images in the songs we introduced them to. Still, every now and then the boys' awareness of adult music caused a problem. One of our sons, when he was playing with his father at the park, was invited to join a Christian-themed group of parents and preschoolers called God and Me. When the group gathered into a circle, the leader asked each child to name his or her favorite song. My son and husband listened as kids called out titles like "Jesus Loves Me," "Mary Had a Little Lamb," and, yes, "Wheels on the Bus." When the group turned their attention to my son, who in that particular moment of his life was especially enjoying the music of Queen, he blurted out, "Fat Bottomed Girls!"

Now that they're all teenagers, the boys make their own playlists, and each year on my birthday I can usually count on receiving at least one carefully curated collection. I love that they take the time to think about me and my own musical preferences (which more and more are much different from their own) and choose songs they know I'll like.

So play music for your kids because, yes, it can benefit them in many ways. But do it as well because it's fun, and because it gives you one more way to bond with them.

Nipple Confusion

Nursing mothers may need or want to use a bottle or a pacifier at times. Will switching from the breast to the bottle interfere with your baby's breastfeeding routine? Can a bottle or a binky lead to "nipple confusion" that could disrupt or prematurely end your baby's desire to breastfeed?

Competing Opinions

Perspective #1: Using a pacifier, and switching back and forth from breast to bottle, can make it difficult for your baby to latch onto the breast. Since sucking from a bottle is easier for babies, they may refuse to take the breast when you want them to return to it.

Perspective #2: Once breastfeeding has been established, your baby won't have difficulty switching from breast to bottle and back again. In fact, since there may be occasions when you can't breastfeed your baby, it's a good idea to familiarize your child with a bottle. And pacifiers can be extremely effective at helping babies soothe themselves.

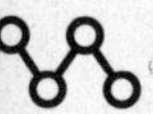

What the Science Says

EXPERTS AND STUDIES disagree regarding even the existence of nipple confusion. As one recent article put it, "Even with the increased focus on breastfeeding, it remains unclear to researchers, clinicians, and parents alike if and to what extent using an artificial nipple (pacifier or bottle nipple) negatively impacts breastfeeding outcomes and practices."

Still, we can draw certain conclusions. A 2015 review of fourteen articles on nipple confusion and its effect on the "efficacy/success/duration" of breastfeeding found emerging evidence of nipple confusion related to the use of bottles, but "very little evidence to support nipple confusion with regards to pacifier use." Nipple confusion does exist, in other words, but primarily in the case of bottles, not pacifiers.

Lactation experts generally accept this conclusion and therefore advise nursing mothers to wait until babies are three to four weeks old before introducing the bottle. The reason is that breastfeeding is more challenging than drinking from a bottle, so it's best to wait until nursing is well established before offering the easier alternative.

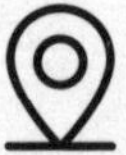

The Bottom Line

NIPPLES COME IN different shapes and sizes, as do babies. Some infants won't have any trouble with nipple confusion and will be able to switch back and forth, using a bottle and a pacifier without any real effect on nursing. But since that's not the case for all babies, ideally you would wait to introduce the bottle until breastfeeding is well established and your infant has "mastered" the art of nursing by being fed exclusively at the breast.

That said, nursing moms, you've got to take care of yourself as well. If you need sleep or a break, if you're dealing with mastitis, or if there's another situation where it makes more sense to have a co-parent or another caregiver bottle-feed, then you might decide to explore that alternative. After all, ongoing sleep deprivation can lead to more serious risks than nipple confusion—for example, depression, illness, or a car accident—and it can keep you from feeling sane or being the kind of mother you want to be. Doing what's ideal for your infant shouldn't come at a cost to your physical or mental health, since what's truly best for your baby is to have a healthy mom.

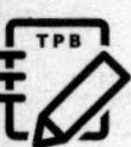

On a Personal Note

I WISH I'D known this when I had my first baby. For one thing, I would have been more open to sharing the feeding load after the first few weeks. Then, I would have been more open-minded about pacifiers. With my first, I was so worried in his early days about latching on that while I did eventually turn to the pacifier in desperation—and it was a real soother for him—I would have been a lot less worried about it. With my next two, I was less of a worrier overall and knew that usually things work out, so I was willing to use the bottles and pacifiers when it made sense to do so.

n

Nursing Baby to Sleep

Newborns will practically always fall asleep once their belly is full. As babies get older, though, mothers have more say in whether they let them fall asleep while breastfeeding. Are there problems associated with nursing a baby to sleep? What benefits does it offer?

Competing Positions

Perspective #1: Getting into a habit of nursing your baby to sleep is fraught with potential problems. For one thing, if he develops a habit of nursing to fall asleep, he could wake up in the night needing to nurse at every little arousal. Instead, he needs to learn to self-soothe. Also, babies who fall asleep at the breast may become distraught when they wake up in a different environment, alone. You should therefore rouse your infant before putting him down.

Perspective #2: Nursing your baby to sleep provides the closeness that's so crucial for bonding. It's a memorable, soothing, and sleep-inducing experience, typical in cultures all over the world. It's not abnormal, not some sort of bad habit that you'd be creating.

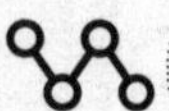

What the Science Says

THERE ARE TWO key points to emphasize here. First of all, whatever you decide about actually nursing your child to sleep, make sure that he's nursing at some point in the evening. The research shows that nighttime breast milk contains nutrients that aid in sleep and are vital for your baby's physical and cognitive development. Tryptophan, for instance, is a sleep-inducing amino acid, and evening breast milk contains a greater amount than milk accessed during the day. Also, tryptophan is "a precursor to serotonin, a vital hormone for brain function and development. In early life, tryptophan ingestion leads to more serotonin receptor development." This serotonin leads not only to more favorable sleep-wake cycles but also to improved brain function and elevated mood. What's more, even the act of sucking results in the release of a hormone called cholecystokinin in both mother and baby, producing a feeling of sleepiness.

Rousing your baby before putting him down in the evenings won't rob him of any of these benefits. This research simply speaks to the importance of nighttime breastfeeding.

But is there anything wrong with allowing babies to fall asleep at the breast? The AAP weighs in with a resounding yes, warning mothers not to nurse their babies to sleep because doing so can create unhealthy sleep patterns. The same goes for allowing infants to doze off while drinking from a bottle. The concern, according to the AAP, is that babies will get the message that they're unable to go to sleep without drinking milk. Parents should therefore "try not to use the breast or bottle as a sleep pacifier."

The AAP's position is based on a good deal of evidence. Some sleep experts even consider falling asleep while breastfeeding a sleep disorder, since it causes problems with babies waking in the middle of the night, unable to return to sleep. Studies have consistently found that babies who are put into the crib already asleep are more likely to wake up and need to be comforted to return to sleep, whereas those who are put to bed still awake are typically better at self-soothing and going back to sleep without parental assistance.

It's worth noting, however, that many researchers and other authorities worry about the physiological and psychological toll on upset babies who aren't comforted because their parents are following rigid, strictly imposed sleep-training (or other parenting) methods. One scholar writes that "typically, babies don't adjust to such regimens without experiencing transitional distress. And even those who advocate sleep training for babies warn that 'cry it out' methods are inappropriate for babies less than 6 months."

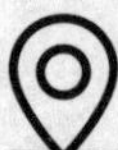

The Bottom Line

THE MAIN SCIENCE available on this question has to do with how bedtime breastfeeding might affect the baby's (and thus the parent's) wake-sleep cycle. This research does support the claim that nursing babies to sleep *can* delay or interfere with their ability to develop good sleep habits. However, other factors are at play. You might decide that the joy, intimacy, and peacefulness of nursing your baby to sleep outweigh the risk of getting less sleep due to more frequent nighttime wakings. Or that since it's the quickest way to get your baby to sleep, it allows you more time for self-care, or to have time with your other kids or your partner, and that it works best for you and your baby.

You may feel that nursing your baby to sleep for the first few months is the best way to go, particularly if you have a really sleepy child who's difficult to wake after nursing. You may at some point decide to nurse mostly to sleep, then rouse your baby slightly so that he's making the final transition to sleep by himself, and you incrementally work toward the goal of his falling asleep from an awake state. Just remember that you may need to keep revising what works best in your home, to get the most amount of sleep for everyone concerned.

On-Demand vs. Scheduled Feeding

With babies, especially newborns, it can seem as if they want to eat *all the time*. That's why some people advise parents to feed their infants on a schedule of two- to four-hour intervals, arguing that on-demand feeding (also referred to as "continual feeding," "on-cue feeding," or simply "demand feeding") can have detrimental effects. Should you let your baby eat on demand, or is it better to set up a schedule?

Competing Opinions

Perspective #1: Babies have tiny stomachs and need to feed often. Sometimes they even need to "cluster feed" during growth spurts. Follow your infant's cues when she's hungry. Doing so has long-term benefits in terms of growth, health, breastfeeding success, and even cognitive development and IQ.

Perspective #2: We should obviously follow a newborn's cues and allow her to nurse whenever she's hungry. Soon, though, babies need a schedule, which not only is more convenient for the parent and the rest of the family but also allows everyone to get better sleep, since the child learns to eat at regular times during the day. One especially concerning result that could be associated with on-demand feeding is that it has the potential to lead to obesity, since by definition it means allowing babies to eat whenever they want.

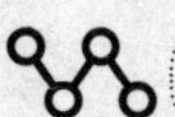

What the Science Says

WHILE MORE RESEARCH is needed, the available science argues conclusively for on-demand feeding over restrictive or scheduled feeding. As the AAP puts it in a flyer regarding healthy childhood weight, "You provide, your child decides." The logic behind the approach, borne out by research, is simply that babies should be allowed to tell us how much milk they need and when they need it. If we don't respond to their needs, they can become dehydrated or remain hungry, particularly during certain growth spurts. On the other hand, if we follow their lead, they'll end up getting just the right amount.

And it's not just about the right amount. It's also about the symbiotic relationship between mother and child. Women's breast milk varies in terms of calorie and fat content, and infants are all different; plus, what a given baby needs in terms of energy requirements will vary as the baby grows. Scheduled feeding doesn't allow very well for these changing dynamics. Demand feeding, on the other hand, supports the feedback loop that allows the mother's body to know how much milk to produce and the baby's body to receive what it needs.

These benefits appear to apply to both breastfed and formula-fed infants. The concern that formula-fed babies tend to consume more calories and therefore need more controlled, scheduled feedings has not been borne out by the scientific evidence. Both sets of babies have been shown to adjust their intakes as needed, whether they're drinking breast milk or formula.

As for practical outcomes related to on-demand feeding, the benefits are numerous. Especially with preterm babies, demand feeding is associated with improved breastfeeding success, growth, health, and psychological adjustment. On the obesity question, several studies have refuted the claim that demand feeding will lead babies to overeat and develop weight problems. Most research reports either no link at all or a higher likelihood that restricted and scheduled feeding will lead to higher body weights.

One other pair of research outcomes worth mentioning—maternal well-being and children's cognitive development—were examined in a long-term 2013 study that found a correlation between scheduled feeding and both higher levels of maternal well-being and poorer cognitive and academic outcomes for children. In other words, scheduled feeding was found to lead to parents who slept better and were happier and more confident, but with the trade-off that their children did less well on IQ tests from ages five to fourteen years. The authors emphasize that while the maternal outcomes aren't necessarily causal—"perhaps mothers who were getting more sleep or felt more confident were more likely to initiate and succeed in establishing a schedule"—the results concerning the cognitive abilities of the children could be chalked up to causality.

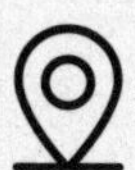

The Bottom Line

SCHEDULES AND ROUTINES help us live our lives and order our world. But when it comes to interacting with a breathing, living human being, we have to be very careful about becoming rigid. And when we're talking about newborns, we have to set aside many of our own individual desires and even needs, within reason, in order to provide what they need. This is one of those times. Sure, it'd be great if we could count on feeding an infant every three hours throughout the day and then putting her down for the evening. But this is one more case where being a parent means letting go of our need to be in total control, and instead being responsive to our children and giving them what they need, when they need it—at least for this early part of their life.

Sometimes fear of spoiling children creeps into this conversation, and as children get older it's important that we remember that need is different from desire. But you can rest assured that providing what your infant needs and wants does not translate into her becoming a spoiled child. Later you'll provide limits, boundaries, and rules (see the entry "Discipline") that give your child practice handling the disappointment from not getting her way, but for now, feed your baby when she communicates that she's ready to eat. You can trust her.

As your infant grows and matures, both you and she will settle into routines that make life at least a bit more predictable. But for now, when it comes to feeding (and so many other things), pay more attention to your baby than you do to the clock.

Organic Clothes and Bedding

The "green movement" has been expanding into the world of parenting and involves not only feeding babies organic food but outfitting the nursery with organically produced products for the crib and closet. Should you go organic to protect your baby?

Competing Opinions

Perspective #1: Organic clothes and bedding don't contain chemicals that can come into contact with babies' skin or be inhaled, meaning they'll be likely to cause less irritation and health problems. Also, products grown organically are better for the environment.

Perspective #2: There's no evidence of any health benefits in using organic clothes and bedding. Since they're more expensive, harder to find, and available in fewer colors, there's no reason to make this commitment.

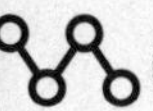

What the Science Says

IT'S UNDERSTANDABLE THAT parents are increasingly concerned with protecting their infants' skin and lungs from chemical residues present in conventionally produced clothing and bedding. Overall environmental awareness continues to grow as well, and plenty of parents are motivated by the idea of purchasing products that haven't been produced with the use of pesticides and processes that can be harmful for water and wildlife.

When it comes to whether conventionally grown fibers will affect your baby's skin and overall health, though, the science simply isn't there. No studies support the claim that there are scientifically proven health benefits to using organic products, or that nonorganic products are unsafe in some way.

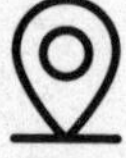

The Bottom Line

YOU MAY DECIDE, for ideological or environmental reasons, to go organic when you choose your baby's crib sheets and pajamas. But if you're looking for a research-based rationale that says your child's health is at risk if you use conventionally grown products, you're not going to find one.

That doesn't necessarily mean there's no reason to buy clothes and bedding made of organic cotton. It just means that science hasn't *found* a reason (and there may not be one). Especially if your child is susceptible to allergies or easily irritated by chemical exposure, or you're just more comfortable with organic, you might decide to avoid the risk that comes with potentially harmful compounds. If it matters to you and you can afford the additional expense, why not? But based on what we know, there's no real reason to worry about the standard clothes and bedding friends share with you or that you can pick up wherever you like to shop.

Organic Foods

According to the USDA, consumer demand for organically grown foods now accounts for 4 percent of total U.S. food sales, and that number continues to rise, with three out of every four traditional grocery stores offering organic products. Should responsible parents prioritize organic meals for their infants? Is it really better for the health and safety of a baby?

Competing Opinions

Perspective #1: Feeding your baby organic foods will offer her better nutrition and limit her exposure to potentially harmful chemical pesticides, antibiotics, and growth hormones. Doing so will also be better for the environment and for local farmers and communities.

Perspective #2: Nonorganic foods are just as nutritious as organic, and since the government sets safe limits on chemical residues, there's no difference in health concern. In fact, there are health-related reasons *not* to feed your baby organic foods, since doing so will limit her exposure to and tolerance for chemicals that are present in most foods she'll eventually encounter. Beyond all that, conventional foods are less expensive.

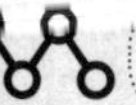

What the Science Says

IT'S NOT EASY these days to filter through all of the political and scientific complexities to get a clear read on where research comes down on organic foods. In 2012, the AAP conducted what it called an "extensive analysis of scientific evidence surrounding organic produce, dairy products and meat." The review's specific conclusion makes two different statements that may sound a bit counterintuitive. On one hand, evidence doesn't exist that an organic diet will lead to better health or a lower risk of disease, or that organically grown food contains more nutrients (vitamins, minerals, antioxidants, proteins, and lipids) than nonorganic food. The AAP doesn't deny the possibility of added nutritional value in organic food and milk; it just says that research hasn't proven the point.

On the other hand, studies have found that organically grown vegetables have lower pesticide levels, and meat from organically raised animals has a lower probability of being contaminated by drug-resistant bacteria. Whether or not these data are statistically relevant—and whether these factors actually make a difference for overall health—is still to be determined. The USDA, which verifies organic food to ensure its authenticity, follows suit, making no guarantees about the nutrition or safety of organic items. And another 2012 study discovered lower levels of contaminants in organic foods, but again found no convincing evidence that they prevent health problems.

Each of these studies and reviews, in other words, essentially found that despite the fact that conventionally grown foods contain more contaminants than their organically grown counterparts, there's no scientific evidence that eating organic foods will actually make a person healthier.

In 2016, a report for the European Parliament performed another review of existing research—381 entries appear in its references section—and offered conclusions that differed slightly from the AAP's 2012 report. Like the AAP's document, the European report also found, for the most part, a lack of compelling research regarding the health benefits of organic food. It did determine, however, that the prevalent use of antibiotics in the raising of livestock contributes to "the development of antibiotic resistance in bacteria—a major public health threat because this resistance can spread from animals to humans." This report advocates for organic farms where antibiotics are restricted and animals are allowed to roam in natural conditions, thus lowering the infection risk,

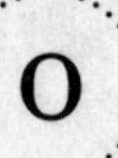

"with potentially considerable benefits for public health." The report also points out certain potential dangers associated with pesticides, including their effect on children's IQ when the mother was exposed to foods produced from pesticides during pregnancy. As one of the study's authors put it, "Although the scientific evidence on pesticides' impact on the developing brain is incomplete, pregnant and breastfeeding women, and women planning to become pregnant, may wish to eat organic foods as a precautionary measure because of the significant and possibly irreversible consequences for children's health."

The other key dynamic typically discussed in this debate is the environmental impact of organic farming. Research has compared conventional, nonorganic farming to what's called alternative farming practices, which include reducing the use and effects of synthetic fertilizer and pesticides, promoting species biodiversity, and more fully implementing organic management of crops. These studies have shown that conventional farming with pesticides has the potential to harm soil, water, and local wildlife. Organic farming, on the other hand, promotes biodiversity, reduces exposure to pesticides for both human and nonhuman populations, protects water supplies, and uses less energy while producing fewer greenhouse gases.

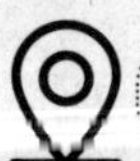

The Bottom Line

IN THE ABSENCE of reliable longitudinal studies, the beneficial lasting effects of an organic food diet are still unclear. However, some feel comfortable following an "ounce of prevention" philosophy in lieu of a proven "cure," especially when it comes to babies and their developing bodies and brains. Keep in mind, though, that you'll typically pay more at the checkout for this ounce of prevention. Some estimate that consumers pay 10 percent to 40 percent more for organic foods than similar conventionally produced products, with certain products going for a much higher premium. And if you have to drive a long way to get to a market offering organic options, this will impact the overall cost as well.

In the end, while ironclad evidence is lacking regarding the nutritional advantages of organic products, the environmental benefits, along with the absence of synthetic growth hormones in organic foods, may leave you wanting to watch for ways to get them into your baby's diet to some degree. If you can afford to buy organic, you can play the odds that they might offer these advantages, including a decreased exposure to toxins. If your family can't manage the additional expense, you can still feel good that a well-balanced diet of conventional, nonorganic foods contains all of the nutrients your kids need.

Pacifiers

What are the risks and rewards of using pacifiers? Is it better to avoid them altogether?

Competing Opinions

Perspective #1: Sucking is instinctive during the first few weeks of life, and it can have a soothing, calming effect that allows babies to regulate themselves and relax when they're upset. It can also help them sleep and even reduce the risk of sudden infant death syndrome (SIDS). Plus, it helps babies avoid becoming thumb suckers, and even if pacifier use becomes a beloved habit, it'll be easier to eliminate than thumb sucking.

Perspective #2: You need to be really careful with pacifiers. They can create confusion when it comes to breastfeeding, and there's an increased risk of ear infections, dental issues, and speech problems. Overreliance on pacifiers might cause you to miss cues that your baby is hungry, and it can interfere with sleep, since an infant can become dependent on the pacifier, resulting in middle-of-the-night crying spells if it falls out.

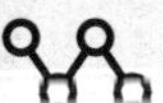

What the Science Says

RESEARCH SHOWS THAT the very act of sucking offers legitimate benefits. The AAP lists pacifiers as one aspect of a method for pain relief in newborns and infants undergoing minor procedures. Another study has found that "non-nutritive sucking" in preterm infants is associated with shorter hospital stays and improved bottle feeding.

It also appears that there's no credible science showing that pacifiers will keep you from breastfeeding successfully. Various reviews of pacifier use in healthy full-term infants have found that it had no impact on the

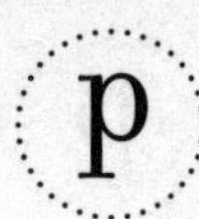

continuation of breastfeeding. Still, since there are questions regarding some of the methodology of these studies, the AAP cautions against beginning pacifier use too early, since it might interfere with the establishment of successful breastfeeding.

Perhaps the biggest benefit offered by pacifier use is the role it plays in the prevention of SIDS. Research is clear in finding a strong association here. The AAP therefore recommends that parents offer pacifiers to their infants at the onset of sleep "after breastfeeding is well established, at approximately 3 to 4 weeks of age."

Despite these benefits, there are genuine drawbacks to pacifier use as well, with studies showing that the use of pacifiers may increase otitis media, or middle ear infections. However, these infections occur *less often* in babies under six months old, when the SIDS risk is highest. In addition, one study demonstrated that sucking in general—pacifier use, thumb sucking, or a combination of both—is what is correlated with earaches and certain other illnesses, not specifically sucking on pacifiers. Still, the AAP recommends weaning children from pacifiers relatively early, encouraging the limiting of pacifier use at six months to moments when the child is falling asleep, and terminating pacifier use around the age of ten months. The American Dental Association and the American Academy of Pediatric Dentistry are a good bit more patient, discouraging pacifier use after four years of age.

Other negative outcomes are associated with using a pacifier for too long. Normal pacifier use during the first two to three years doesn't cause long-term dental problems. However, prolonged use risks misalignment of teeth. Use beyond the age of three may produce noticeable negative changes that become more severe after five years. As for whether a pacifier impacts speech development, research hasn't shown that correlation. Investigators have hypothesized that such a relationship might exist, but the closest research has come to demonstrating it is to suggest that the presence of a pacifier in a baby's mouth might prevent him from babbling and imitating sounds and thereby produce a delay in learning to speak; it might lead him to be less interested in communicating orally at all.

One other interesting and potentially negative consequence worth mentioning relates to emotional development. Research has suggested the possibility that when pacifier use is extended (over three years), it can disrupt the "facial mimicry" ability of a male child. (These results were not found in female children.) The basic idea is that a pacifier in the mouth may prevent a young child from mimicking the facial expressions of the people around him, which keeps him from developing a proper understanding of the nuances communicated by those expressions. Extended pacifier use therefore predicted lower emotional intelligence and a limited ability to take someone else's perspective. A related study found that adults were less accurate in assessing and resonating with children's emotions when a child was using a pacifier. Why these results were not seen in girls is speculative. The primary theory is that adults may talk about feelings and emotions more and be more emotionally expressive with girls, so female children get more practice building emotional literacy.

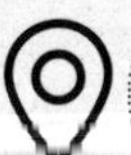

Bottom Line

EXCEPT IN UNUSUAL circumstances, there's no compelling reason to actively discourage pacifier use, especially from three to four weeks through the first six months of life, when it can be particularly beneficial. Some experts warn that risks begin to outweigh the benefits around six to ten months and increase even more notably after two to three years.

If you worry about having to break your child of the habit when he's older, try using alternative soothing behaviors such as swaddling, rocking, singing soft music, and infant massage. But babies need to be comforted, and if a pacifier allows your child to self-soothe by sucking, and nothing else seems to help, then by all means hand him a binky.

If your child gets really attached to the pacifier and it's a tool that works well for your child to practice emotional regulation, plan to wean him over time, starting with its use only during sleep or occasionally in the car, and then get rid of the habit by replacing it with another soothing object.

On a Personal Note

ONE OF MY sons was such a pacifier connoisseur that he may have crossed over into hoarder territory. He slept with one in his mouth and one in each hand. When he was two and it was nearing the time to graduate beyond the pacifier stage, we started playing a game where he'd throw his "paci" back into the crib after he woke. We'd say, "You stay there, paci!" and it would remain in the crib until the next bedtime. Eventually we had a "Bye Bye Paci" party with a cake and candles, and we clapped and even sang those words to the tune of "Happy Birthday." After the singing and clapping, we had him put all the pacifiers into a box to "share with the new babies who need pacis." (Don't worry, we didn't really give used pacifiers to anyone.)

I was so worried this would be traumatic for my son that I kept the pacifiers in the back of the closet for a while, just in case. He did indeed cry and ask for them for a few days. But we told and retold the story about the pacifier party and helping all the new babies who didn't have any, and within a week they were a distant memory. I remember thinking that if I'd known saying goodbye to pacifiers would be that painless, I would have done it sooner.

"Parentese" and Baby Talk

What some call baby talk—now more typically referred to as "parentese speech"—is the communication style many of us tend to use automatically when we speak to babies. We address them almost musically, exaggerating our words and drawing out vowels while speaking in a higher pitch. (Instead of "Look at the dog," we might say, "Oooo. Look at the doggiiie!") Does this approach help infants learn the patterns, rhythms, and vocabulary of their native language? Or would it be better to speak to them "as an adult"?

Competing Opinions

Perspective #1: Speaking to your infant using an "adult" tone will model language more correctly than parentese. Using baby talk with infants dismisses how intelligent they are and misses out on opportunities for them to learn at a higher level. It could potentially cause them to learn infantile patterns of speech that will be difficult to unlearn.

Perspective #2: Speaking to your baby in parentese will help your baby acquire the patterns of her native language more easily. She'll pay attention more when you speak and will therefore learn the grammar and vocabulary associated with language. There's a reason talking this way comes naturally.

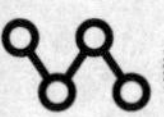

What the Science Says

THERE'S NO AMBIGUITY here. The use of parentese has been studied for decades, and the results are clear. Across languages and cultures, and controlling for socioeconomic status, it aids a child in terms of attention and social responsiveness, vocabulary acquisition, spoken word recognition, vocalization, and on and on. Babies even prefer parentese over standard speech.

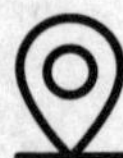

The Bottom Line

"PARENTESE" APPEARS TO be a language that most of us—parents, caregivers, family, and friends of all ages—are universally and naturally fluent in. And, according to research, that's a very good thing for infants who are setting out on an amazingly rapid journey of primary language acquisition. You don't have to make up baby babble, saying things like "goo goo ga ga." And it may not feel natural right away. But just speaking to your newborn using elongated vowels and a higher-pitched melodic tone will capture her attention and allow her to more easily hear and imitate the sounds of her language. As she gets older you'll obviously (we hope!) move toward standard speech. But for now, let her have fun learning the patterns, rhythms, and vocabulary of her language while interacting with you in a way that connects you two even more.

Pets

Many parents (and soon-to-be parents) have a pet whom they consider part of the family. In fact, 63 percent of households with infants under twelve months have at least one family pet. When an infant is introduced into the home, should new boundaries be established to protect the health and safety of the child? Can pets be a beneficial influence on an infant's development?

Competing Opinions

Perspective #1: Even beloved family pets can be unpredictable and pose a danger to your newborn or infant. The sweetest pooch could conceivably step on a baby or scratch them in the face with its paw. Pets may even have infections that can be transmitted to babies. Be very careful if you decide to allow a pet to spend time around your infant consistently.

Perspective #2: Having a pet is one of the best things you can do for your baby. It actually makes kids smarter to be around animals. Healthier, too. On top of all that, the child will be happier in a home with a pet.

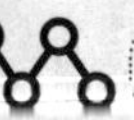

What the Science Says

IT'S DIFFICULT TO overstate how beneficial it is for children to grow up with pets as members of the household. The American Academy of Child and Adolescent Psychiatry, in its 2019 statement on pets and children, put it this way: "Developing positive feelings about pets can contribute to a child's self-esteem and self-confidence. Positive relationships with pets can aid in the development of trusting relationships with others. A good relationship with a pet can also help in developing nonverbal communication, compassion, and empathy."

Aside from these intra- and interpersonal benefits, studies also show that being around pets leads to significant health advantages, primarily in terms of lowering the risk of obesity and allergy-related maladies. Researchers have also found that exposure to cats and dogs in the home can contribute to infants' cognitive development—possibly due to increased opportunities to read and scan the animals' faces—as well as their overall happiness and well-being.

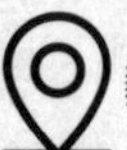

The Bottom Line

MORE RELATIONAL, HEALTHIER, smarter, happier—it's hard to argue with those outcomes. Pets can provide comfort, company, and entertainment to the family. But use your common sense and pick a safe pet. If Fluffy isn't so nice and fluffy and instead becomes aggressive and unpredictable, then the benefits won't be worth the risk.

Even when you've determined that the animal is safe, commonsense care should be taken to shield your infant from a pet who might not want the attention of a curious infant at a particular moment—that wagging tail can be awfully tempting, and your dog or cat might not be keen to have it tugged. Be aware, as well, that as kids become mobile a pet might view them differently, so make sure to keep an eye on the interactions. Also, take precautions to avoid access to a cat's litterbox and other pet-related items that can do harm.

One other consideration is timing. Taking home a newborn will be demanding enough without having to deal with all that comes with raising a puppy, so maybe you don't want to take on both challenges simultaneously. But as long as you're using reason, being safe, and considering timing, then introducing your baby to the family pet can lead to a happy and rewarding relationship for both of them.

Getting a family pet is not something you have to do, of course. If animals aren't your thing, it's not at all crucial that you go straight to the humane society to rescue a furry friend. But the science is clear that if you already have a pet or you'd like to add one to your family unit, your child will likely reap all kinds of advantages.

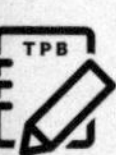

On a Personal Note

I LOVE DOGS. I grew up with them and I love having them as part of the family. Scout, Moby, Jasper, and now our beloved Bluebell: our boys have grown up with these four dogs, and the benefits have been seemingly limitless. Through having pets they've learned to be responsible, yes. Walking the dogs, picking up poop, feeding them, even giving one of them a bath after she was sprayed by a skunk (and then, I kid you not, having to repeat the process two weeks later when it happened again!)—these are just some of the ways my kids have gotten practice being reliable and conscientious.

But beyond this, they've had more objects for their love. As I write this sentence, my youngest son is working on solving a Rubik's cube on the couch while Bluebell rests her head in his lap. Yesterday on the way home from school, Blue heard a siren and began howling out the open car window, leading to laughter from all of us in the car, along with the motorcycle guy waiting next to us at the red light.

Each new opportunity to love and care for another living thing opens up a child's heart that much more, preparing the child to live a life full of empathy and relationship.

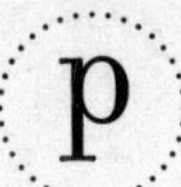

Postpartum Depression

How do you know if you're suffering from a perinatal mood disorder, particularly postpartum depression?

Competing Opinions

Perspective #1: Most women who have recently given birth can feel down from time to time. It's perfectly normal to feel depressed. Postpartum depression is rare, so don't worry too much about it. Be patient. You're probably just trying to figure things out right now.

Perspective #2: It's true that most women will experience some form of postpartum blues, but that's different from actual postpartum depression, which can be debilitating and seriously affect not only you but also your relationships and your child. It's actually somewhat common. If you think you might be experiencing some of its symptoms, seek help right away, as intervention can make a huge difference.

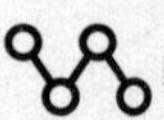

What the Science Says

RESEARCHERS ESTIMATE THAT anywhere from 60 percent to 80 percent of women will experience what some call the "baby blues," which produce mood swings, irritability, anxiety, reduced concentration, and a general sense of feeling down. These symptoms can last for a couple of weeks after childbirth.

Postpartum *depression* (PPD), on the other hand, can manifest in some of the same signs and symptoms, but they'll be significantly more severe and long-lasting. (If they last longer than two weeks, then it's likely more than the blues.) PPD can leave the mother feeling completely debilitated and, when severe and chronic, can even hinder a baby's physical, mental, and emotional development by interfering with the bond between mother and child. In extreme cases, it can even endanger the life of the mother or that of her baby, since suicide and infanticide are both potential dangers associated with PPD. In the most extreme cases, which are quite rare, women experience postpartum psychosis, where they suffer from paranoia, delusions, hallucinations, and more.

It's estimated that between 8 percent and 20 percent of new mothers in the United States suffer from PPD, so it's not at all an uncommon experience. In fact, maternal depression is considered the number-one complication related to pregnancy and childbirth. The baby blues are generally less severe, are shorter in duration, and don't interfere with your basic functioning, including tending to your infant. PPD, though, can leave you struggling to perform activities of daily living. A quick online search can show you indicators to watch for, but here are a few to pay attention to: losing interest in activities you typically enjoy; having trouble bonding with your baby; withdrawing from family and friends; doubting your ability to care for your child; having thoughts about harming yourself or your baby.

The good news is that for 90 percent of women, PPD can be treated with medication or a combination of medication and psychotherapy. Even breastfeeding is still a possibility while you're on some antidepressants. Some women elect to quit breastfeeding when they go on these medications, but before you do so, discuss the question with your doctor. You may be able to continue nursing even as the depression is being addressed pharmacologically. (For information about specific medications as they relate to breastfeeding, see the NIH LactMed Drugs and Lactation online database.)

Some researchers point to what's called paternal postpartum depression, by the way, where new fathers experience symptoms such as sadness, fatigue, anxiety, and sleep disorders. This especially occurs in men who already have a history of depression or are struggling financially or in their relationship.

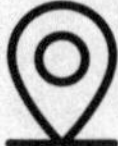

The Bottom Line

YOUR OB/GYN SHOULD be screening for PPD and other perinatal mood disorders in your postnatal checkups, and many pediatricians will do so as well. The AAP encourages pediatricians to assess maternal mental health, and many states now require Medicaid to cover screenings. But you can't count solely on a doctor discovering potential issues. Unfortunately, many doctors never bring up the subject, so it's important that you pay attention to what's taking place in your body and mind in the weeks after your baby is born.

If you recognize PPD symptoms in yourself, you're not alone. Many women experience PPD. This is simply part of your birth experience. It's not pleasant, I know, but it's now part of your story, and it's crucial that you address it immediately. As soon as you begin noticing warning signs, talk to your ob/gyn, primary care physician, pediatrician, and/or mental health provider. The vast majority of moms who suffer from PPD can be treated successfully, go on to full emotional health, and thrive alongside their child. The sooner you speak up and seek support, the sooner you can begin feeling better, more fully connect with your baby, and enjoy your new role as a parent.

If you're having thoughts about harming yourself or your baby, get help immediately. That may mean enlisting the help of your partner or a family member, or even calling 911 or your local emergency number.

If you're reading this as the partner or loved one of a person who seems to be suffering from PPD, keep in mind that she may not be able to recognize that she's depressed. She may tell you she's fine, but once you see red flags, resist the temptation to wait to see if things improve. Many women don't realize they have PPD until later, and wish they'd known and been able to get some support. So seek medical attention immediately.

Potty-Training an Infant

There are alternative approaches to getting a child "toilet ready" (see the entry "Elimination Communication"), but for our purposes here, I'll discuss what's traditionally understood as toilet training: preparing a child to transition from the diaper phase into the stage where he uses the toilet or a portable potty, which then can be emptied into the toilet.

The big question for most parents is about when to begin the process. There's a fairly sizable amount of research on the subject that can help guide (and/or confuse) you as you make the decision for your child and your family. It does appear that in the United States, almost all toddlers (98 percent) can maintain a dry diaper during the day by the time they're three years old, whereas by the age of two, only about a quarter (26 percent) achieve what's called "daytime continence." Many parents, understandably, want to ditch the diaper as soon as possible. But how early is too early to begin training?

Competing Opinions

Perspective #1: The best practice is to wait, even as long as twenty-four months, before attempting to toilet-train your child. Potty training during infancy (birth to twelve months) can be a frustrating experience for both of you and will likely take much longer than if you wait. It might even cause psychological or behavioral problems. And it can definitely lead to lots of vexation on the part of the parents when the process isn't successful in a fairly short amount of time, giving the baby a bad experience before there's much success.

Perspective #2: Lots of other cultures know that early toilet training is not only possible but that it offers several advantages. It helps prevent diaper rash and other infections and eliminates the prolonged need for diapers, meaning you're being both more economical and more eco-friendly. It also offers you the option of earlier education for your child, since many nurseries and preschools require that kids be free of diapers. Plus, you won't have to go through that phase when the diapers are heavier and especially noxious, and the accidents much more distasteful to clean up.

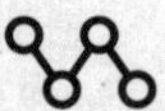

What the Science Says

BEGINNING THE TOILET-TRAINING process early—before the age of two, generally speaking—does offer certain advantages. For one, those kids are more likely to be out of diapers sooner. The process itself is likely to take longer overall, but at least you'll be done with it. Also, urinary tract infections, which often result from failing to completely eliminate all bacteria-containing urine, are less common in kids who are trained earlier. So that's a reason for beginning sooner, especially if your child is prone to urinary tract disorders.

However, there are persuasive reasons to wait a bit longer before beginning the process. One study shows that children who begin toilet training earlier than two years of age are three times more likely to develop problems related to what's called "dysfunctional voiding," like daytime wetting and constipation, when compared with children trained later. The lead researcher of that study explains that those issues are largely caused when kids try to hold their poop and pee, which he explains is "essentially the definition of potty training." So when kids are too young to understand the importance of elimination, it's more likely that they'll "hold it" and face the health consequences. This study is contradicted by another, however, which states that earlier training is *not* associated with constipation or stool withholding.

It's also possible to wait *too long to begin training,* according to research. The dysfunctional voiding mentioned earlier is not unique to toddlers; if toilet training is initiated later than thirty-six months, many of the same problems, especially constipation, are more likely to crop up. And a late starting age can increase the risk of problems having to do with infections and incontinence.

As you can see, there are potential negative consequences associated with starting too early or too late. That's why one group of researchers has suggested that there's a "magic window" for beginning training around the age of two. The AAP takes a similar position: "There is no right age to toilet train a child. Readiness to begin toilet training depends on the individual child. In general, starting before age 2 (24 months) is not recommended. The readiness skills and physical development your child needs occur between age 18 months and 2.5 years."

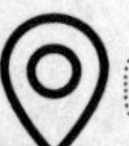

The Bottom Line

WHETHER THERE'S A "magic window" or not, the best thing you can do is to look for "toilet readiness" if your child is around age two. Can he follow your directions and understand the general idea? Can he stay dry for at least a couple of hours at a time? Can he read his own body's cues? If so, he's probably ready. The idea is to make the decision considering what's developmentally appropriate for your child so that his toilet-training experiences are positive and successful enough to prevent him from avoiding the toilet even more. Make the choice that helps him feel positive and confident about his emerging independence in the world and joining the ranks of those who use the big-kid potty.

If your child is younger and you want to give it a go, the most obvious benefit you'll enjoy is that he will likely be in his big-kid pants sooner. Keep in mind, though, that the research definitely shows that beginning the process sooner increases the time it takes before you'll see success.

So that's not a bad way to boil it down: Would you rather have your child out of diapers sooner but undergo a longer and potentially more frustrating process, or would you prefer to wait and have it be a bit quicker and less challenging overall?

Either way, young children should never be punished for having an accident or not eliminating in the toilet. If parents are harsh, punitive, or negative, it can backfire, making the child fearful of using the bathroom, which then makes the toilet training even more challenging. Be positive, available, and encouraging, and your child will learn to use the toilet when they are developmentally ready.

Probiotics

Some foods and supplements include—naturally or by design—live microorganisms that are reputed to produce health benefits. These microorganisms are called probiotics. Because of these anticipated benefits, probiotics have become a billion-dollar industry that continues to grow worldwide. Are they safe to give to babies? Do they lead to better health and wellness?

Competing Opinions

Perspective #1: Probiotics replenish your child's "good bacteria" and help the body function properly. They are harmless and exist naturally in many foods, offering benefits related to a baby's skin, gut, and brain.

Perspective #2: We don't know enough about probiotics to give them to babies at this time. There's a chance, of course, that they might do some good, but there's also the possibility that they could cause harm and lead to health problems down the road. It's best to be cautious and avoid them.

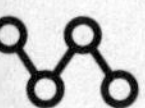

What the Science Says

RESEARCH ON PROBIOTICS in general shows some promising results in terms of improving health. But authorities and investigators consistently caution that persuasive evidence is still lacking. For one thing, defining exactly what's meant by the term "probiotics" isn't always easy, in a scientific sense, given that it refers to such a broad subject—live microorganisms that can aid in healing and health. Since there are so many different categories of probiotics, including different types of bacteria, and so many ways that various manufacturers produce and market them, reliable research is hard to come by. Not only that, the wide variety creates problems for governmental oversight agencies, since the products fall under assorted regulatory bodies with varying requirements about demonstrating whether a product is safe and effective.

A 2019 document from the National Institutes of Health explains that as a result, "the U.S. Food and Drug Administration (FDA) has not approved any probiotics for preventing or treating any health problem. Some experts have cautioned that the rapid growth in marketing and use of probiotics may have outpaced scientific research for many of their proposed uses and benefits."

When it comes to the benefits of giving probiotics to babies, the scientific community is even less confident. Some studies have published findings indicating that probiotics produced negative results in terms of infant health. One study even found that "probiotic exposure during infancy has limited effects on gut microbial composition yet is associated with increased infection later in life."

Yet several other investigations show positive outcomes in terms of producing good effects relating to skin disorders, colic, diarrhea, and even neuropsychiatric disorders. Still, even these studies contain, almost without exception, some version of the old "but these results are preliminary and will need to be replicated" line. What's more, there are so many different strains of probiotics, and they work so differently on different children according to their ages and stages of life, that it's difficult to say with certainty how much good they will actually do once they're turned into commercial products.

Because of this uncertainty, organizations including the AAP, the WHO, and the Committee on Nutrition of the European Society of Pediatric Gastroenterology, Hepatology and Nutrition have all called for more research and/or oversight before they will conclude that probiotic products are safe and effective for children.

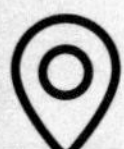

The Bottom Line

IN A FEW more years, we may have a reason to give our youngest children probiotics, confident that they will be building gut health, or preventing eczema, or warding off other maladies. Or we may determine the opposite. The point is that right now, we just don't know for sure. The research isn't there, nor is the ability to adequately regulate probiotics as commercial products. Therefore, if you're curious, or inclined to explore the possible benefits probiotics may offer, talk to your trusted pediatrician with this information in mind. Otherwise, this is one item you can cross off your list.

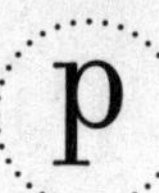

Pumped Milk vs. Direct Breastfeeding

With close to two-thirds of American women now working outside the home, using pumped breast milk has become a major part of breastfeeding in the United States. What advantages does direct breastfeeding offer over feeding a baby using expressed milk? Are there any drawbacks, aside from convenience?

Competing Opinions

Perspective #1: Using pumped breast milk is a healthy alternative to feeding at the breast. It's a nice option for working mothers and those who don't want to breastfeed in public or at certain events, and it offers independence for those times when the mother needs a break, is experiencing pain, or has to be away from her baby. By expressing milk, caregivers can better regulate the timing of feedings as well as share day and night feeding duties. If the baby needs to gain weight, a parent can better measure how much milk the baby is ingesting. In addition, mothers can pump after feeding at the breast to increase their milk production and build a surplus supply.

Perspective #2: Using pumped breast milk rather than nursing at the breast means mothers miss out on certain benefits that come with breastfeeding their infants directly: skin-to-skin bonding opportunities, convenience, health advantages, and more effective soothing when children are upset. Breastfeeding allows baby and mother to more effectively have their systems of production and hunger in tune with each other, which will help production and supply keep up with the baby's needs.

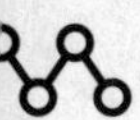

What the Science Says

BOTH PERSPECTIVES ARE right: expressing milk really is a great alternative, and direct breastfeeding does offer some definite advantages. For one thing, nursing directly can promote a mother's recovery from childbirth, since it causes the hormone oxytocin to be released into her body. The hormone causes a contraction in the uterus, thus reducing postpartum bleeding. Direct breastfeeding offers other benefits regarding the amazing symbiotic relationship between mother and child. When the baby's saliva interacts with the milk at the breast, it sends signals to the woman's brain regarding what nutrients and antibodies the baby needs at that particular stage of his life. Plus, the mother's breasts are assessing the supply of milk the baby needs, where more breastfeeding communicates that more milk needs to be produced, so the infant has enough supply, but the mother is not creating a surplus beyond what's needed.

It's also the case that milk can become contaminated with bacteria if it comes into contact with pumps and containers that haven't been cleaned thoroughly. Not only that: while stored breast milk offers many of the same nutrients of milk direct from the nipple, it loses benefits the longer it's stored. Many moms will store the breast milk in the freezer, which is perfectly fine when following milk storage guidelines. But studies have found that the process of freezing, thawing, and heating the milk can degrade the proteins and vitamins typically present in fresh breast milk.

One other factor to consider has to do with the skin-to-skin connection that takes place when breastfeeding. Obviously, a mother will have numerous other opportunities to bond with her child every day, even if she doesn't nurse directly at the breast. But the intimacy of a breastfeeding moment between mother and infant really is a powerful relational interaction. Plus, mothers who nurse will tell you, and research has confirmed, that nursing at the breast is a great way for babies to experience relief from distress or pain, as when they receive their vaccinations.

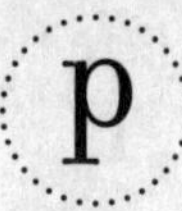

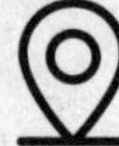

The Bottom Line

YES, THERE ARE definite advantages that come when a baby nurses directly from the breast, so do it when you can.

If you're a mom who works away from your child, take advantage of opportunities to nurse when you have the opportunity—evenings, mornings, weekends, or whenever you're free. You should be applauded for doing the hard work of pumping and still providing your infant with the benefits of breast milk for the hours you're away.

Also, knowing the benefits of direct breastfeeding shouldn't preclude mothers who aren't working outside the home from pumping milk and finding occasional, even regular, opportunities to get a break. After all, let's face it: as wonderful and beautiful as it is, breastfeeding can be an all-consuming activity that can be tiresome and make us feel less like women and more like functional mammals. We all need a break at times, and feeding expressed milk is an excellent way to get a breather. Plus, it gives siblings, grandparents, and especially a non-nursing parent a chance to have the intimate bonding experience of feeding the baby while holding her close.

So if you have the option and inclination to breastfeed, do it. But both direct nursing and offering pumped breast milk offer extensive health and nutrition benefits. The costs, convenience, and lifestyle of the caregivers will all factor into the decision to nurse your baby at the breast, to pump, or to use a combination of both.

Reading to Baby

Is it really that important?

Competing Opinions

Perspective #1: Yes, it is.

Perspective #2: Agreed.

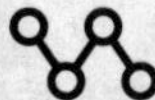

What the Science Says

DO IT. As much as possible.

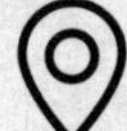

The Bottom Line

DO IT. Then do it some more. As often as you can. There's no debate, and aside from safety, love, and good nutrition, it might be the best gift you can give your baby.

S

Screen Time

With the ubiquity of screen devices, how much is too much for infants? Can TV, videos, phones, and other screens be beneficial for a child's development? Can infants actually learn from them? Or should you focus exclusively on human interactions and active play for at least the first few years of your child's life?

Competing Opinions

Perspective #1: The recommendation of the American Academy of Pediatricians—that children under two completely avoid media with the exception of occasional video chats with family members—exists for a reason. Screen time for infants and toddlers correlates with cognitive, developmental, and speech delays, as well as negative health issues and even lowered academic success. You can't escape screens entirely; they're everywhere. But as much as possible, keep them from becoming a routine part of your kids' world. Instead, play and talk with them to develop skills related to language, physical development, cognition, and relationships.

Perspective #2: The AAP provides excellent advice on a number of subjects and should be relied upon as an authoritative voice on children and their health. On this issue, though, they're simply not being realistic. There's a plethora of age- and content-appropriate media these days, and it might even give a child the benefit of being more technologically savvy in our high-tech world. And even if the video is less educational and merely entertaining, how is that a bad thing? Let's be honest: virtually all parents need a break from time to time, and screens can provide it. Obviously, we have to be careful not to overdo this. But like it or not, we're all digital citizens now, and avoiding screens until a child is two is simply not feasible for modern parents.

What the Science Says

DESPITE THE AAP'S recommendation (with which the World Health Organization agrees, by the way), 68 percent of kids younger than two use screen media in a typical day, with an average of over two hours per day. And this is *direct* exposure to the digital world. Beyond that, younger children also often encounter hours more of "background" or secondhand screen exposure, such as a television or other screen being on while someone else is watching or simply as background noise.

But is this really a problem? Research says yes. First of all, there's practically no evidence that children under the age of one learn language or conceptual skills via a screen. Actual intellectual and linguistic abilities develop as a result of interactions with a live caregiver. The reason is simple. Developmentally, infants don't have the memory and attentional skills, or the symbolic understanding, necessary to learn from two-dimensional images the way they do when interacting with actual humans and the physical world around them. While some value may be derived from observing a two-dimensional world, screen use actually creates what one study calls "a video deficit: reduced learning relative to learning from live and interactive instruction." In other words, the time children spend watching a screen could be better used playing, laughing, moving, or being read to.

Further bolstering the claim that infants and toddlers need live, responsive, face-to-face interactions with actual people is a 2018 study that found that video chatting isn't sufficient to support word learning, even when a live person is on the screen. Researchers found that toddlers were unable to learn the words for various toys while watching and listening to a responsive person on video. The same children had no trouble learning the toy's name when encountering the information through interacting with a responsive person present in the room.

Numerous studies also point to negative health outcomes that correlate with screen time for very young children: sleep disturbances, cognitive deficits, obesity and weight issues later in childhood, language issues, and social and emotional delays. It's important to note that these studies aren't all pointing to causality. In other words, we can't claim that research has determined that digital exposure is the *reason* for these various negative outcomes; it may be that excessive amounts of time in front of a screen simply have an indirect detrimental effect by causing kids to miss the opportunity to be playing and interacting with caregivers and the objects of their world. There are likely other confounding factors as well, and often the studies don't distinguish between types of screens (for example, television versus a tablet) or take into account how stimulating/overstimulating the content might be. But parents should be aware of the correlations between screen time and these negative outcomes, regardless of how confidently we can point to causation or account for the different variables.

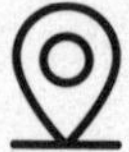

The Bottom Line

THIS ISSUE IS likely going to be a big one for the rest of your baby's childhood and adolescence. As he gets older you'll have to figure out how best to limit screen time and how to protect him from the many dangers it presents—all while taking advantage of the vast number of benefits the digital world offers as well.

Think carefully about this from the very beginning, even when your child is a newborn. You may be tempted to use screens to help regulate your baby's emotions. Infants often calm down when looking at images on a screen. But even though the child may be fixated on the screen—as they may be with a mobile hanging above the crib—the baby can't effectively process information or learn from it. What's more, you don't want to let screens prevent you from learning how to respond to infant distress, and you don't want to give your child the message that every time they're upset or have difficult feelings they should just distract themselves. When parents depend on devices to keep kids calm and quiet, those parents miss out on the opportunity to learn how to handle those moments and build self-efficacy and resilience in their children.

As your baby develops and approaches his first birthday, you'll be faced with the question regarding screen exposure more and more. It may be that you decide to follow the AAP guidelines and avoid any screen exposure at all (again, excluding video conferencing with family members or other special people in your life). If you have a lifestyle that somehow allows for a no-screens-at-all option—either because of your career situation or childcare assistance you have from a spouse or other caregivers—and you find ways to have your child read and sung to and played and laughed with on a consistent basis, then that's obviously going to be more worthwhile than any video, no matter how educational or entertaining.

But most of us don't have that option, and we need a break from time to time. If you're having one of those days (or weeks!) where you haven't had time to eat or sleep or even go to the bathroom, and you feel like you're on the verge of losing it, then putting on *Sesame Street* for twenty minutes might be preferable to the alternative. Be mindful of the content you choose, though. Just because a program is labeled "educational" doesn't mean it's good for your child. When you can, pick content that's created by people who understand child development and kids' brains.

One final note about your baby and screens. Take a moment to consider your own screen usage and how present you are with your child. There's nothing wrong with checking your phone or catching up on recent notifications. But when you're with your child, *be with him*. That doesn't mean frantically and obsessively making sure that every second of every day is totally enriching for your baby, or that you can't just sit back and allow each of you to enjoy some quiet when he's contented. But be aware that our devices have the mesmerizing power to pull us out of a moment and make us less present to the ones we love. Just consider the difference between, on one hand, a mom who's pushing her baby down the street, hears a truck, and says, "Do you hear that big, loud sound? That's a truck! See the big wheels!" and, on the other, the same mom who's reading on her phone and never even notices the noise, much less takes time to interact with her infant about it.

Think, too, as your baby grows, about what you're modeling as a healthy relationship with the mobile devices that are constantly vying for your attention. If you're consistently allowing tech to interrupt interactions, meals, car rides, games, and so on, then that will become your child's vision of normal.

From time to time, you may decide to use your child's interest in a screen to maintain your own sanity. Virtually all of us do. Just keep in mind that in the end, the goal is to be as fully present as possible and engage the attention of your infant, to support his healthy physical and cognitive development by speaking to him, playing with him, and attending to him. Doing so will make it that much easier to read his cues and get inside his mind, making it easier to help him handle moments of distress or challenge down the road.

On a Personal Note

THE STAY-AT-HOME MOTHER of an eighteen-month-old waited to ask me a question after a talk I was giving. She told me she was worried her baby was already addicted to screens. When I told her she could just decide not to give the child a device, she said, "But she'll cry and scream!"

I smiled and assured her that I understood. We want our kids to be happy, and we definitely don't enjoy it when they cry and scream. But often, doing what's best for a child means being willing to let them feel unhappy. We wouldn't let a toddler play with sharp scissors, after all, even if they really wanted to do so. We'd set a boundary, then comfort the child if they were upset about not getting what they wanted. It's the same with screens, I explained.

She said she saw my point. Then she said, "I also think I'm on my device too much. How do you know how much is too much?"

I asked her to think about how much time she was on her device during the day while she was the primary caregiver for her baby. Then I asked, "How would you feel if you hired a nanny to care for your daughter, and that nanny spent as much time on her device as you do on yours?" The mom replied, "I'd fire her."

I have to admit: I really enjoy my phone, and I rely on it heavily. I work from it, I keep up with friends on it, I play music and podcasts on it, I search for recipes on it, and I enjoy my social media. Because of this, I have to remain aware and alert about the example I'm setting for my kids, all of them teenagers now. When they were babies, phones weren't as prevalent, so in our family we've all had to evolve together. Sometimes I think we're doing pretty well in this area, and sometimes I feel like it gets away from us.

I have a few ground rules I've set for myself. Unless it's a rare exception, I'm not on my device right before or after drop-off at school. The moments before the goodbye and after the hello, times that bookend separations, are important opportunities for connection and reconnection. Also—and I'm not always good at this—when I'm with the kids, if I need to reach for my phone, I try to make it conversational and connecting, explaining the purpose of why I'm turning my attention away from them and to the phone. I might explain that I'm wanting to show them a funny video. Or if I'm checking the calendar I'll say, "Let me see what time your basketball game is tomorrow." That way they know that I'm not just checking out of the conversation to scan my Instagram. You can do the same with your baby: "Daddy's going to call Grandma to see what time she'll be here. Do you want to say hi and hear her voice?"

I remember one night when I'd been with our son every second for days on end, without even a solo potty break. My husband saw how frazzled I was, and we both realized that we were missing each other and needed time to connect and to catch up on some conversations. We went to a restaurant, put him in his booster seat, put some headphones on him, and popped in an episode of *Magic School Bus* (which I'd watch repeatedly, even now—I learn so much!) so we could have a glorious, indulgent, twenty-minute conversation. I remember getting a few eye rolls and judgmental stares from others for letting our kid stare at a screen. (It wasn't as common back then.)

The other patrons in the restaurant didn't know about my physical and relational needs, or that I'd spent what felt like six hundred consecutive hours that day trying to provide language-rich, physically active, creative, enriching, developmentally appropriate stimulation (whew!) for my son. What he needed right then—much more than he needed to avoid screen time—was to have a mom who was achieving a rare moment of balance and self-care in her life by claiming some much-needed adult connection.

I often think of that night when I feel judged or when I feel criticism toward other parents arising in me. Those people in the restaurant didn't know my whole story, and I don't know other people's whole story. So maybe we should just smile at other parents and their kids and send them positive, supportive vibes. After all, we're all in the struggle and privilege together, even if we don't all do things the same way.

Security Blankets

Is it OK to let my baby sleep with a security blanket or some other object like a stuffed animal?

Competing Opinions

Perspective #1: Babies can need help sleeping, so if you provide a soft, safe object that can help them feel calm and secure, why not?

Perspective #2: Objects in the crib can be dangerous in numerous ways, leading to choking, strangulation, and other SIDS-related concerns. Don't use them.

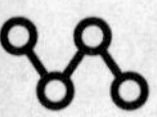

What the Science Says

THE AAP SAYS that for the first twelve months, a baby's crib should be "bare" and free of any soft bedding, bumpers, blankets, and soft toys. Buttons from stuffed animals can become choking hazards, and any type of blanket or soft bedding has the potential to suffocate a sleeping infant.

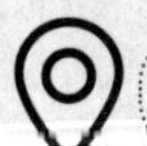

The Bottom Line

THIS IS ONE of those times where less is best. For the first year of your child's life, make sure the crib remains bare and minimal. Even if you find the cutest bumper or stuffed dinosaur you've ever seen, save it for after the first year. Until then, keep the sleeping environment simple and safe.

S

Sedation While Traveling

In case you're making the joke in your head right now, yes, the question is about sedation for the *baby.* Is it a good idea when you're taking a long trip, possibly in the middle of the night? What risks are involved in exchange for the chance of a peaceful flight (or car ride)?

Competing Opinions

Perspective #1: Over-the-counter antihistamines such as Benadryl are harmless and can have a calming effect on a fearful or fussy child. They can also cause drowsiness and make a long trip more peaceful, not only for you and your baby but for the other passengers as well.

Perspective #2: Any medication can have dangerous side effects, and you don't want your infant to experience those ever, but especially not while on a plane or in a car. Antihistamines can cause hyperactivity rather than drowsiness in some children. Look for other ways to make the long trip more palatable for everyone involved.

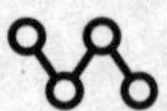

What the Science Says

THE ACTIVE DRUG in Benadryl is diphenhydramine (DPH), which is typically used to treat allergy symptoms. As for its effectiveness in making babies drowsy—for a flight or any other time you need your child to sleep—the science urges caution.

One study from 1976 found that kids ages two through twelve fell asleep more quickly and woke less frequently after being given DPH. But since then, research hasn't replicated those results, with investigators discovering no evidence that DPH enhances sleep quality. A 2006 study, focused on babies six to fifteen months, found not only that DPH didn't improve sleep but also that it possibly "caused low-level hyperactivity in children, thereby negating the sleep benefits seen in some adults." This hyperactivity, sometimes called the "paradoxical effect" of Benadryl and other medicines containing DPH, is often referred to in warnings to parents regarding the downsides of medicating infants to help them sleep.

In addition to the lack of scientific evidence supporting the sedation of infants, we have warnings by health groups and governmental organizations. The NIH, the AAP, and the FDA all discourage the practice, pointing to the paradoxical effect—the possibility that antihistamines and other substances can sometimes create restlessness and agitation.

As with any medication, there are possible side effects associated with DPH, including nausea, headache, constipation, and dizziness. What's more, administering the correct dosage can be difficult, especially given that Benadryl's own dosing guidelines advise against giving it to children under six, or under two for Children's Benadryl. One study shows a link between antihistamine overdose and babies who end up in the emergency room.

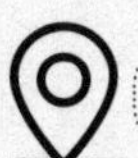

The Bottom Line

THERE'S NO COMPELLING evidence that sedating babies will be effective in getting them to sleep through a long trip. Combine that with possible dangers and side effects, and it becomes a pretty easy decision. Don't medicate your child with the goal of producing drowsiness. There are too many unknowns regarding dosage limits and negative effects to risk the health and safety of your little traveling companion. Having a potentially agitated, hyperactive infant on board is great for funny stories down the road, but in the moment it can be pretty miserable.

Instead, prepare with some books, snacks, and toys, and be ready to sing and get creative to keep your baby happy. (The barf bag on the airplane makes a great puppet!) And letting your child use a pacifier or suck on a breast or bottle can also help alleviate pressure in their ears during takeoff and landing.

Sensitive Babies

Some babies seem especially sensitive regarding stimulation and new experiences: lights, new people, the crush of a crowd, tags on clothes, even the sound of a toilet flushing. Is it better to protect them from what's making them nervous, or expose them to more of it so that they become more resilient and able to handle it in the future?

Competing Opinions

Perspective #1: Babies have to get used to new sights, sounds, and sensations; that's part of growing into their world. We need to be there for them and encourage that growth. We're doing harm when we shelter them from new experiences. Instead, we need to push them beyond what feels comfortable and help them build strength and resilience. Part of loving them is avoiding overprotecting them and helping them grow into all they can become.

Perspective #2: Our first job as parents is to keep our children safe, to help them feel at home and at ease in the world. They're still so little and vulnerable that they require us to shelter and protect them. There will be plenty of time later to challenge them and build resilience. Especially if your baby has a more sensitive temperament, protect him from stressful situations and be patient in figuring out how to help him grow into all he can become.

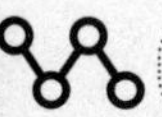

What the Science Says

PARENTS OBVIOUSLY INFLUENCE the way babies perceive and interact with their world. Research backs this up, but it also clearly demonstrates that biological and environmental forces have significant impacts as well.

Your child's temperament, therefore, needs to be considered when you're making parenting decisions. For some temperaments, a particular parenting approach might help; in other kids, the same approach might hurt. In other words, certain parental responses are going to be more effective and beneficial with a child who's naturally inclined to be more shy or sensitive, whereas other approaches will work better with a child who's outgoing and who happily welcomes new experiences.

A huge amount of the research in this area has focused on young children, looking at how their initial temperaments—whether they are high-energy or less so, quick to warm up to new experiences or slow, and so on—manifest as the kids grow older. As you might expect, these studies demonstrate the negative effects of overprotecting children, as well as asking too much of them. And while fewer investigations have focused exclusively on infancy, empirical research on parental responses to sensitive babies suggests that the overall conclusions are consistent with what we've seen in toddlers and preschoolers: "that sensitive and appropriately responsive parenting in infancy is related to more optimal patterns of behavioral and physiological reactivity and regulation." This "sensitive and appropriately responding parenting," in other words, where parents read their children's cues and respond with love and attunement, will typically reduce behavioral problems and help kids be better regulated, both physically and emotionally. The opposite is true as well. A parental lack of responsiveness, especially when it reaches its extreme and results in abuse or neglect, can be related to all kinds of future negative outcomes for children, including impulse control problems, depression, and antisocial behaviors.

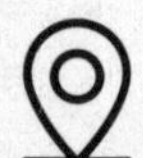

The Bottom Line

WHILE IT'S DIFFICULT to draw causal connections between certain parental behaviors and various childhood outcomes, we can point to patterns that seem well established in the research: primarily, that children whose parents support and protect them, while also allowing them to experience momentary and manageable discomfort without too much stress, have a much better chance of growing into teenagers and adults who, regardless of their temperament, can deal with new and difficult situations without losing control of themselves or their emotions.

When it comes to deciding how much to protect our babies and how much to allow them to grow by undergoing new and challenging experiences, it's like so many facets of the parenting experience: we need to find the Goldilocks sweet spot—not too hot and not too cold. Like older kids and adults, some babies are naturally more disposed to approaching a new situation or input with enthusiasm, and others will be stressed out and automatically avoid it. The goal, with any child, is to provide attuned, sensitive care, reading the baby's signals and figuring out how to give this individual child what he needs in this particular moment.

On a Personal Note

THIS WAS A big struggle for me as a new mom. I had a sensitive, easily overwhelmed baby. When he was about three months old, we traveled to a family reunion. It started off with a drive that took three times as long since we had to keep pulling over because he cried and cried and cried, hating being in his car seat. (I actually think now that he may have been carsick.) And I'll admit, I even somehow contorted my body to nurse him while he was strapped into his car seat as my husband kept driving to get us there. It was a horrid day on the road for us (although one surprised truck driver did get a show).

Once we finally made it to the gathering, my son cried for virtually the whole weekend. Many caring family members volunteered to give my husband and me a break by holding our son, but when we tried it he became even more upset. I even felt pressure to "share" him and let his cousins, uncles, aunts, and grandparents hold him and get time with him. But my instincts told me that much of his unhappiness was *caused* by passing him around amid all the stimuli and noise. I knew we'd have plenty of time later to socialize him, and I felt within my bones that at my son's young age, he needed me to take him to a quieter place, soothe him, and be focused on his needs, so he could know that I would help him feel safe in the world. So I ended up cocooning with him in a back bedroom much of the weekend, and we were both much happier.

Because of his temperament, I made similar decisions not just when he was a baby but throughout his childhood as well. These choices weren't always well received by friends and family members. But I knew I had to deal with my people-pleasing tendencies and build the confidence to step into the role of being less accommodating of others in order to follow my instincts and take care of my kid in the way he needed to be taken care of, even if others didn't agree.

By the way, there were plenty of times, increasingly so as our son grew older, that we found ways to encourage him to face situations that didn't immediately feel comfortable to him. As an infant he needed our protection, but we knew better than to shelter him from every possible challenge as he grew up, and as a result, he's now a highly social young man who's comfortable with himself and has really good people skills (if I do say so myself).

Sign Language

Parenting poses many challenges, one of which is trying to figure out what your baby wants—or, more importantly, needs. Some parents eager to communicate with their infants are turning to sign language, where babies use gestures to tell their caregivers what they're needing or wanting or noticing around them. For our purposes here, when I talk about signing, I don't mean teaching babies American Sign Language or another codified system, but using sign-like gestures with babies to help them communicate with us.

Competing Opinions

Perspective #1: It's a powerful gift to offer a baby, to give her tools by which she can tell her caregivers what's going on in her mind. Long before she has the motor ability to articulate actual words, she can communicate with signs to tell her parents that she hears a train, that she's in pain or afraid, that she wants a drink or another cracker, or that she sees a picture of a fish. Doing so helps reduce frustration for all. Even without a formal program, children can begin to pick up signs and develop a decent-sized vocabulary around the time they turn one. Then, over the next six months, they can acquire dozens of signs, meaning they can tell their parents things their words can't communicate yet. This skill can prove especially helpful to kids with developmental or speech delays, and it can help all children improve their cognitive and emotional development.

Perspective #2: While it's an intriguing idea, baby sign language hasn't been studied enough to risk possible complications that might come with it. What if it delays speech, as babies come to rely on their signs and choose to sign rather than develop and use words? Also, it's not realistic for all parents, since teaching baby sign language requires consistent pairing of the sign with the spoken word, which can be hard to do if your child is in daycare or not with you for hours every day. Plus, while using baby sign language may reduce the baby's frustration at not being able to communicate her needs to her parents, that frustration and confusion will still occur when she attempts to use signs with others.

What the Science Says

SCIENCE IS DEFINITELY inconclusive when it comes to using signs and gestures to communicate with an infant. In a 2000 study, researchers compared two groups of eleven-month-olds, showing that the group that was taught to sign soon became more advanced talkers than the non-trained group. Then, at the age of two, signers showed more proficient verbal skills that were three months ahead of non-signers. At eight years of age, the trained group had IQs twelve points higher than the non-trained group, even though they had stopped signing years earlier. As with any study, we have to look at its specifics, and this one was relatively small, with only 103 infants studied. Still, as the authors pointed out, the evidence at least pointed to the strong possibility "that symbolic gesturing does not hamper verbal development and may even facilitate it." Other research found that the use of symbols and gestures correlated with the later development of social-emotional strengths. These results fell in line with the efforts of speech and language therapists, who for decades have been using different versions of sign language with infants who have speech and/or cognitive impairments.

However, in 2005, a meta-analysis looked at these studies and others and determined that the evidence was inconclusive when it came to whether "teaching gestural signs" actually leads to improved language development. In other words, the review study concluded, we just can't say yet. In response, the authors of the 2000 study defended their conclusions and took issue with the 2005 review finding a lack of positive effects as a result of signing.

Since then, other studies have taken up the question, and over the last few years the argument has continued. A 2014 investigation did find evidence suggesting that "baby sign training had a significant, positive impact on the overall development of the children" observed. That same year, a separate article determined that "while there is no conclusive evidence to support the effectiveness of baby sign intervention . . . there is also no evidence that early exposure to sign language negatively affects typical development."

Some have theorized that parents who decide to use baby sign language may be a self-selected group, in that they may have already given their babies certain genetic and environmental advantages when it comes to language and learning. It might follow, too, that parents who approach their children's language development with this kind of intentionality spend more time reading with and talking to their babies about words and meaning, which in itself could account for a child's increased facility with language or vocabulary later on.

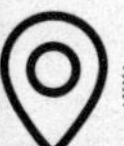

The Bottom Line

WHAT DOES ALL this tell us? Well, at this point there's conflicting evidence regarding whether baby signs offer demonstrable benefits in terms of language development and social and emotional growth. There's plenty of anecdotal evidence of parents (including this one) who are big fans of baby signs, and it's not hard to imagine that introducing babies to the relationship between gestures and words and giving them another tool of reciprocal communication might help them down the road as they learn to talk. But based on current research, we can't conclusively say it does. Even setting aside the question of language and learning, though, there are relational benefits that come with your baby being able to tell you what she's thinking and feeling and seeing. Possessing this tool has the potential to lower her frustration level, to increase communication between you two, and to give you information you might otherwise miss.

Baby sign language is certainly not a "have-to," and you can't count on it giving your child a developmental edge. But if you have the time and inclination, it's a great way to connect with your child, learn what she's interested in and noticing, and let her communicate with you in a fuller manner.

On a Personal Note

WHEN MY GRANDPARENTS learned we were using baby signs, they responded with barely masked skepticism. My grandpa said, "You mean like that gorilla, Koko?" They were worried my kids would never talk.

I assure you that all of my boys talked, on time or early, and developed rich vocabularies. I don't know if learning to sign gave them any kind of cognitive or developmental boost, but I absolutely loved using baby signs. Around ten months, we began teaching our boys just a couple of basic signs—"more" and "done"—from a popular book about baby signs. Then, once they got those two down, we added more. By the time our eldest was fourteen months, he knew more than sixty signs, many of which we just made up intuitively. That means that between eleven and fourteen months, he learned to articulate dozens of concepts, words, and ideas that he didn't yet have the motor ability to say.

While it makes sense to me that this process would benefit a child's language-acquisition process, my favorite part of teaching signs was that I got to communicate with my sons earlier than I typically would have. Signing allowed me to see what caught their attention and what they were interested in. For example, I remember reading *If You Give a Mouse a Cookie* to my son when he was about a year old. At one point I turned a page, and my son started signing the word "lawnmower," which involved pretending he was pulling the cord to start a mower. I said, "Lawnmower? Where?" He pointed at the page, and then I saw a mower in the back corner of a shed. It excited us both to have joined in this moment, and without the signs it wouldn't have happened—and I wouldn't have known that the lawnmower was interesting to him.

Even more helpful, we taught our sons to sign "hurt" (hand on the forehead like we're checking for a fever) so they could tell us when they felt pain. They learned "scared" (patting the heart with the right hand, like a heart beating fast), which then morphed into "need comfort," so they could let us know when they were upset or scared. Our sons would make up their own signs, too, which was really fun and sometimes funny, like when one son made a sign for "mama's milk" by emphatically slapping his own chest.

I know what the science says, but I wouldn't trade the signing months with each of our boys for anything. I think it let them realize early on that we wanted to know them and listen to them and to build trust, that we "got" them and would respond to their needs. Our family still uses a couple of signs to this day, even though the boys are all in their teens and taller than I am now. We all still do a soft, right-handed fist to pound twice on our heart to communicate "love you" when they're about to get on a plane or say goodbye.

S

Silence vs. Noise in the House

Issues of hearing loss (given that babies often have fragile ears) and ensuring sound sleep will mean managing noise in a household. Is using white noise a good idea?

Competing Opinions

Perspective #1: If you, as an adult, hear a noise that bothers you, you can typically turn down the music in the car or cover your ears. Not so for babies. They have to rely on us to protect them from uncomfortable or harmful sounds. This includes toys and white-noise machines designed to promote sleep by producing ambient noise to mask other sounds. All of these noisemaking devices are potentially dangerous.

Perspective #2: You need to protect your baby's hearing, but a certain amount of noise is actually desirable, especially if there are other children in the house or the child will be going to daycare soon, where he'll need to sleep while surrounded by other children and the clamor they create. If he is used to sleeping only in silence, any little sound will have the potential to wake him. Give him enough environmental noise to get used to sleeping in a variety of settings.

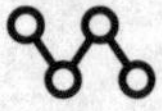

What the Science Says

ACCORDING TO THE American Speech-Language-Hearing Association, sounds at or below 70 decibels (dBA) are safe. Normal conversation is typically thought to be at about 60 dBA. But what's called sensorineural hearing loss can take place when we're consistently exposed to noise that's at or above 85 dBA. For infants, the AAP recommends limiting noise levels in hospital nurseries to 50 dBA.

Aside from the actual volume of the sound, distance from the noise and length of time exposed to it can also contribute to how damaging it can be. People talk about the "three Ds": decibels, distance, and duration of noise.

Research has shown that many baby toys can be excessively loud, and this is especially problematic in that babies often like to hold toys close to their ears. One study looked at ninety different toys marketed for babies six months and older and found that eighty-eight of the ninety had a mean noise amplitude of 85 dBA. Even when held 30 cm away, nineteen of the toys still had a noise amplitude greater than 85 dBA. (According to the National Institute for Occupational Safety and Health, this amplitude would be dangerous even for adults if they were exposed to it for more than eight hours at their job.)

Even sleep machines can be far too loud. An AAP study found that out of fourteen infant sleep machines, all fourteen produced sound at above the recommended 50 dBA level. Three of them produced levels greater than 85 dBA. The authors of the study pointed out as well that the devices were sold with limited or no instructions for how to use them safely. The investigators therefore suggested placing the sleep machines as far from the infant as possible, setting the volume on the lowest possible setting, and limiting the duration of use.

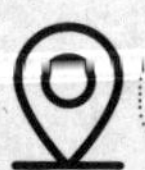

The Bottom Line

BABIES' EAR CANALS are smaller than adults', and their skulls are thinner, meaning that noise has the potential to do more significant harm and result in noise-induced hearing loss. A child's inner ear and hearing nerve can be damaged if he is exposed to extremely loud noises or if he is around loud noises for long periods of time. It's therefore our responsibility, as parents and caregivers, to limit the decibels, distance, and duration of noise our children are exposed to. This can apply to toys we give them, music we play for them at home or in the car (especially since car seats may be right next to the rear speaker), movies we take them to see, and yes, even the sleep machines we put in their rooms. So remain aware of noises in your baby's environment.

As for establishing your baby's sleep habits, you have to do what suits your household and your lifestyle. As always, consider the temperament and preferences of your child, as well as what his environment is likely to be. It might be necessary to make sure that various sounds are a part of the home environment since he will need to get used to sleeping in the absence of silence. But protect his hearing and remain connected to his ever-changing desires and needs.

Sleep Training

Helping your baby sleep regularly—and, ideally, through the night—has tremendous benefits for both of you. But what's the best way to make that happen? Some people swear by sleep training, and others worry that it will cause harm to the infant, the parent-child relationship, or both. How do you maximize sleep for your whole family while building trust and strengthening your relationship with your baby?

Competing Opinions

Perspective #1: Sleep training offers numerous benefits, the primary one being increased sleep for the whole family—which is important for everyone's physical and emotional health. There's no evidence that, assuming parents are emotionally attuned, their babies will suffer any negative effects of sleep training.

Perspective #2: When babies cry, it's a signal of distress or discomfort, letting us know they need help. When you don't respond to your infant's request for help or comfort, you're communicating that when she needs you, she can't count on your being there.

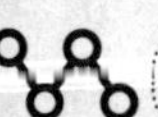

What the Science Says

AS YOU TURN to this entry in the book, you're likely wondering whether it's OK to sleep train. You might be hoping that the science "allows" it, or maybe you're dreading that research will tell you that it's the best thing for your baby and your family. But what is it that we're really talking about? What do we mean when we talk about sleep training?

Let's start by getting clear on terms. Sleep training is *not* synonymous with the harsh "cry-it-out" approaches, where babies are fed and diapered, then placed in their cribs and told good night, not to see their parents again until morning. The idea behind this strategy is that infants are allowed to "cry it out" and thereby become trained to sleep on their own. The most famous proponent of this method is Richard Ferber, who once wrote that even if a baby becomes so upset that she vomits in the crib, parents should still resist picking her up. Instead, they should quietly clean up the mess and quickly leave the room so that the training can continue. As one leading researcher on infant sleep puts it, this more severe cry-it-out approach "is not usually recommended nowadays because of the distress it causes parents and infants." (For the record, Ferber later revised and clarified some of his more controversial positions, explaining that he does not endorse "simply leaving a child in a crib to cry for long periods alone until he falls asleep." He also softened his position on co-sleeping and took a more flexible stance on other child-rearing subjects.)

So if modern, attuned sleep training isn't about setting the baby in the crib then turning off the light and listening to her scream until she wears herself out, what is it? And what does research say about it?

Among current authorities and experts, "sleep training" is often used as an umbrella term for many different types of strategies for helping babies learn to fall asleep on their own. Just by keeping lights dim while we change a newborn's diaper before bed, we're beginning the process of sleep training, teaching the baby to understand that we sleep at night. Other strategies call for slightly rousing the infant after he's nursed or bottle-fed to sleep so he has to complete the process of dozing off in the crib on his own. Or the parent might remain close to the crib, possibly even placing a hand on the baby, or sleeping in the room near the infant, slowly moving farther away over time (a process sometimes referred to as "camping out") while helping the child learn to relax and go to sleep on his own. Some even consider co-sleeping a type of sleep training. (See the entry "Co-sleeping.")

For our purposes here, when I discuss sleep training, I'll be referring to an approach that involves putting the baby down while he's still awake but growing sleepy, then waiting a period of time before responding to his cries. After an interval, the parent responds and offers reassurance and comfort. Then the interval is extended a bit more, and the process is repeated until the baby falls asleep. The goal is that after a few nights of this progression, the baby becomes comfortable enough with the new arrangement to go to sleep on his own, and then sleeps better when he does. This approach is still known by many as "Ferberizing," and there are more and less gentle and nurturing ways to practice it. Since the harsh and rigid versions, again, aren't recommended by most experts and authorities on infant well-being, this discussion will examine the science surrounding the gentler versions, where parents do allow their babies to cry as they develop the ability to fall asleep by themselves, but the parents remain emotionally connected along the way.

(As a caveat, by the way, I'll offer a quick reminder that this isn't a how-to book. If you're looking for specific strategies and instructions, you'll find many valuable books and websites that will walk you through various approaches in a step-by-step manner. Here, I'm simply offering a broad, global perspective on how this particular approach to infant sleep is currently viewed among researchers who study the subject. My hope is that it will help you get an overall feel for whether you want to sleep train your baby, and help you explore many of the relevant variables as you make your decision.)

Research on sleep training exists, but not as much as you might expect, given its importance. There aren't more than twelve to fifteen strong, high-quality studies available on sleep training and its outcomes, and even in these, researchers are often examining multiple strategies in the same study, typically relying heavily on parental report, which is quite open to bias. Further, studies that compare various sleep strategies to one another are rare. As a result, we should be careful about drawing conclusions too confidently. Still, we can discuss the scientific opinions and findings regarding the primary questions surrounding sleep training: Is it effective, will it harm the child, and will it damage the parent-child relationship?

In response to the first question, research responds in the affirmative. Sleep training does appear to improve sleep for both child and parent. This enhanced sleep leads to reduced parental fatigue and improvements in mood, including diminished parental depressive symptoms and marital conflict, all of which play significant roles in child outcomes. It's better for the baby's sleep as well. One study looked at caregivers who used gentler sleep-training interventions and found that five months after implementing the strategies, the number of parents reporting sleep problems had dropped by nearly 30 percent. The conclusion of another study emphasized emotional responsiveness on the part of the parent, explaining that "parents' emotional availability to children in sleep contexts promotes feelings of safety and security and, as a result, better-regulated child sleep." The news isn't all good, though. Other studies have found that many of the sleep-related gains experienced early on as a result of sleep training will wax and wane over the following months. Science warns us, in other words, not to expect that sleep training is a once-and-for-all moment in our child's life, not to believe that we're somehow pressing the "perfect sleep" button that results in nighttime bliss for the remainder of childhood. Still, at least on a short-term basis, sleep-training techniques do seem to offer sleep benefits for a majority of babies.

But does it harm the child in some way, to allow her to experience moments of stress or being upset as she falls asleep? One thing seems clear: any improved sleep helps in the short term. Research has found that babies who sleep better can be more adaptable, better emotionally regulated, and less easily distractible.

Still, some parents worry about the stress caused by sleep training, even when it's done in a nurturing fashion (as in the "camping out" method or other gentler sleep-training approaches). For most babies, short-term, mild-to-moderate stress can actually be positive in terms of building resilience, and tolerable stress experiences lead to what's called stress inoculation. The fear, however, is that allowing especially upset babies to cry too long will establish a pattern of stress activation that leads them, especially those who are more sensitive and easily dysregulated, to develop *less* resilience over time. There's concern that for babies who have a stress response that's extreme, frequent, and long-lasting, the physiological and psychological distress may be harmful.

The argument is that a cessation of crying might not be evidence that the baby has learned to "self-soothe," but instead that she has instead *adapted* to the stress by shutting down, even possibly dissociating to some extent, employing a defensive strategy that triggers what one researcher calls "an enduring hypometabolic state that might be problematic for the high-energy needs of the developing sleeping brain." Indeed, research has demonstrated higher nighttime levels of the stress hormone cortisol in very young infants (one to three months) when mothers are less "emotionally available" during the times associated with sleep. (This study looked at mothers, but, likely, the same would apply to fathers as well.)

A related study measured the levels of the stress hormone cortisol in both babies and mothers during a sleep-training experiment. The researchers found that after two nights of crying it out, infants stopped expressing their distress by crying, but their cortisol levels remained at the same elevated level. Without the infant crying, the maternal cortisol levels decreased, even though the babies were experiencing the same amount of distress. The worry is that during the sleep-training process, parents are being conditioned to believe that everything is all right, when in actuality babies have simply learned to stop crying and go to sleep, even though they're still upset. Other research, by the way, has shown that children in distress don't always cry, depending on the circumstances and the child's temperament.

The cortisol study has been criticized for certain methodological limitations—chief among them that baseline cortisol levels weren't clearly established—and we should be careful about interpreting the results as evidence that sleep training is harmful for babies. But it makes sense that this study's results would at least lead to further and improved research on the question, since it raises the possibility that a sleeping baby isn't foolproof evidence that sleep training is successful across the board. After all, waking through the night is part of typical development for infants and young children, as is the need for the comfort and support of their parents. Those who challenge the efficacy of sleep training therefore raise the concern that children who learn not to cry at night have actually learned not to ask for or expect comfort, even when they're internally distressed and need help.

Just how much stress an infant experiences during sleep training has not been well studied. But we do know that babies have a wide range of hardiness, sensitivity, and need, and that the intensity of the stress will be different for different babies. In other words, some babies might get highly distressed being left to cry for five minutes, whereas other babies might experience only mild distress.

Certain researchers have attempted to examine the question of sleep training's effect on overall well-being by looking at children years after the fact. Some studies have found no negative outcomes resulting from sleep training in terms of overall child behavior, even up until age five or six. In one of the most robust studies to date, researchers followed up five years later on children who had undergone some sort of "behavior-modification program designed to improve infant sleep." The study concluded that there was "no evidence of longer-term adverse effects" on children's mental health, including their behavior, stress levels, sleep, or their relationship with their parents.

For what it's worth, by the way, this study also didn't find any longer-term *positive* effects, either. Put differently, it's not an endorsement of sleep training, and for those uncomfortable with the idea, the study doesn't argue that all parents *should* sleep train. It simply found that caregivers don't have to worry that gentler sleep-training techniques will do long-lasting damage.

What about the parent-child relationship? Will a baby who's been sleep trained lose overall trust that her parent will attend to her needs? Some studies have shown that sleep training either has no effect on the parent-child relationship or can even improve infant security and attachment. The key, according to many researchers, is the emotional availability of parents in the process, which can be correlated with improved sleep in infants. At the moment, there's no evidence that gentle sleep training, when approached with an emphasis on honoring the child-parent bond, will negatively impact the degree of closeness in that relationship.

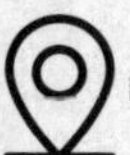

The Bottom Line

TO SUM UP: Does the science say it's OK to sleep train? Yes, as long as you remain emotionally attuned to your child. Does research say you *should* do it? No. Just as there's no definitive research establishing that sleep training is directly harmful to babies, neither is there proof that it's beneficial. The truth is that, as far as we can tell given the body of research at this point, it doesn't make much difference at all in terms of long-term effects on a child. As is so often the case, this decision comes down to your feelings about what you, your child, and your family need right now.

To explain a bit more fully: You might choose to sleep train simply because it makes the most sense to you and appears to be the best choice for your family. Your situation may leave you with little choice, either because of a work schedule or some other family dynamic. If you do sleep train, make sure to educate yourself on the least-stressful and most relationship-honoring methods available. For one thing, most experts agree that you shouldn't start too early, suggesting waiting until your infant is four to six months old, once good feeding habits and sleep patterns have been established. Also, keep in mind that babies should never be left in highly stressed states for long periods of time. The "rule," according to whichever expert/approach you're following, might call for allowing your child to cry for three minutes (or five or ten or more). But there's no scientific data about the amount of time a caregiver should wait before responding to a cry. Some infants might calm down and be able to fall asleep more quickly with shorter intervals of parental comfort, and some might calm down more quickly with a bit longer. As you've heard me say throughout this book, you should consider the information at hand, then, based on your knowledge of your own child's needs—which change all the time throughout development—let your instincts guide you to make the best decision possible.

Keep in mind, too, that there's a big difference between an intense "attachment cry" from a highly stressed baby who is in distress for long periods of time, and a mild "fussy cry" from a baby who isn't really stressed but is just trying to get settled and who falls asleep fairly quickly. When stress ceases being mild and tolerable and turns intense and toxic, it can create distrust and fear rather than building resilience. As a result, the baby can be left unsure about whether, when she is in distress, anyone will come. So if your baby fusses a bit, doesn't get too upset, and then puts herself to sleep, fantastic. That's likely a valuable resilience-building experience. But every baby is different, and they have different needs at different times. I believe that if a baby is in intense distress for long periods of time, that's not healthy. In that case, she *needs* a parent to help her feel soothed and safe enough to go to sleep, at least at that time in her development.

One key point if you decide to sleep train: be sure to check your expectations. Babies typically aren't great sleepers. They have raw little nervous systems and small stomachs, and as a rule, they just can't sleep through the night early on. Plus, even when a baby begins sleeping well, illness, developmental spurts, separation anxiety, teething, travel, or another change can crop up to affect sleep, and you may have to start over. Remember that sleep training isn't a one-time event that means your baby will always sleep through the night. That likely won't happen for years. Even healthy, well-adjusted school-age kids can regularly wake in the middle of the night and need to be comforted by their parents. You'll likely be working on sleep for a few years, any which way you go. Plus, for many babies—some estimate as high as 20 percent—no amount of sleep training will be effective. So be careful with any assumptions that you'll be able to find the "right" program that leads to blissful slumber throughout the household.

If you decide *against* any formal sleep training, take care of yourself so that you can be the parent your child needs you to be. It's always a difficult balance to strike, deciding just how much of ourselves and our own needs to sacrifice for the good of our baby. If you determine that it just doesn't feel right to let your infant cry at all, and you choose to forgo sleep training, find a way to get enough rest so that you'll be capable of showing up in the various ways your infant needs.

My final bottom-line reminder on this subject is that every child is different, as is every family. Each child will go through different phases, and a given approach might be effective during one stage but not in another. It's therefore essential that you remain attuned to your baby's needs and prepared to flexibly adjust to what's called for in each new moment. Your needs matter, too, and your sleep is important. Make decisions based on what your child requires, considering your own needs and those of other family members as well. Listen to experts, but follow your own instincts and be willing to adjust when circumstances change and call for a shift in terms of what it means to best care for your child and yourself.

On a Personal Note

I HEARD ARGUMENTS in favor of various cry-it-out methods when I was a young mother, but as someone who had studied physiological states of stress and the role of the attachment system in modulating stress, I just couldn't get comfortable with the idea. I had lots of friends who believed in and practiced some version of crying-based sleep training (some harsh, some gentler.) They were loving, attuned, intentional parents whom I respected. Some of their stories made me jealous. ("My baby fussed just a little for the first night, almost not at all the second night, and now we're all sleeping! It's changed our lives!") Some of their stories, I'll acknowledge, made me feel judgmental. ("My baby screamed her head off for over an hour until I finally went in, and she had vomited all over her bed. I'm not sure if she's actually sick or just got that upset.") One friend said, "She needs to learn that if she cries, I'm not coming." And I felt deeply that I wanted my baby to learn the opposite of that message. So, I read about every version of sleep training, from the strictest to the gentlest, but I just couldn't feel at ease with any approach where I had to let my babies cry without responding. The way I saw it, if my priority during daytime hours was to respond when my children needed me, I wanted to do the same at night. So for the most part, my husband and I chose not to use any type of approach that involved letting our babies cry.

Looking back now, was it the correct decision? I think it was, for me and for our family. From one perspective, I took the easy road, at least in the short term. I nursed my babies to sleep because it was the quickest avenue to freedom each evening and the fastest way back to sleep in the middle of the night. Plus, our firstborn was a sensitive baby who got stressed easily, so I felt that allowing him to cry would overwhelm him.

But I'll also admit that my babies weren't great sleepers, so I was exhausted a lot, and at times I was pretty frustrated and tired, even resentful about having to nurse at 3 a.m. (and again at 4:30). It's also the case that I was a stay-at-home mom during most of that time, and I had a husband with a job that allowed him to get up with our kids first thing in the morning so I could sleep a bit more. I tried some gentler methods and they didn't seem to make much of a difference, but I didn't know about the "camping out" method, and I think I would have been comfortable trying that. But I would have also followed my instinct to go to my babies if I felt that they were needing my presence to feel safe, and to settle.

In the end, I don't regret responding to my babies when they called, day or night, and I'm confident that knowing myself, I would have regretted letting them cry without support. I wanted them to know that if they were communicating "I need you," I would come. But it was a big sacrifice, and my husband and I paid a price for it. Who knows—maybe our children did, too, in that they might have slept better if I'd sleep trained, and they would have had a more rested, more patient mother. For what it's worth, my boys were all good sleepers by the time they were two or so—and they're making up for all those lost hours of sleep now that they're teenagers who like to sleep a lot! And, my friends who used cry-it-out methods also have awesome kids and great relationships with them. So, every family has to do what feels right to them and what works best for everyone involved. If I had another baby now, I'd still be pretty uncomfortable not responding when she cried. But after looking back, I'd be fine with allowing her to mildly and briefly fuss, to give her an opportunity to fall asleep on her own.

S

Sleeping in Car Seats, Swings, and Strollers

Is it safe to let a baby sleep in a car seat or some other "sitting device" like a swing, bouncer, or stroller?

Competing Opinions

Perspective #1: For some babies, it seems that the only way they'll go to sleep is in some sort of device. If you have to use a swing, stroller, or car seat to get your infant to sleep, by all means do it. Your child needs his sleep, and so do you.

Perspective #2: Babies die every year while strapped into sitting devices. It's not smart to let babies sleep in sitting devices for long periods of time in situations where the caregiver might not realize that the child is in danger. It's fine if you put your baby in a car seat while you're driving, but get him out once you arrive. Same with your stroller. Even if he wakes up when you move him, that's better than taking a risk.

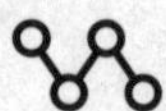

What the Science Says

WHEN TRAVELING IN a car, make sure your baby is in a properly installed car seat. There's no question about that. (See "Car Seats.")

But the car seat shouldn't be used in place of a firm, flat crib. According to a 2019 study published by the AAP, there's a real danger in allowing an infant to sleep for long periods of time in a sitting device like a car seat. The ten-year study, which looked at almost twelve thousand infant sleep-related deaths, found that 3 percent of those deaths occurred in sitting devices, most often involving car seats. That might sound like a small percentage, but it's big enough to be considered significant, and it's definitely significant to those families who lost their babies.

A primary danger is asphyxiation. Especially when a car seat is improperly used, its straps can get wrapped around a baby's neck and lead to strangulation. An infant's airway can also be blocked when his head rocks forward, since young babies often don't have the neck strength to lift their heads. The other key danger highlighted in the study occurs when sitting devices are set on elevated surfaces and fall, or on a soft surface where the device can tip over and lead to suffocation.

Authorities including the AAP and the CDC continue to firmly advise that babies be placed on their back to sleep at all times, both for napping and overnight.

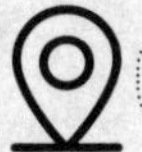

The Bottom Line

BABIES ARE GOING to fall asleep in car seats, swings, and other devices. That's perfectly fine. What matters is that you avoid leaving your child to sleep there, and that you keep a watchful eye on them. It's tempting to take a nap yourself or grab a quick shower, but health authorities repeatedly warn that babies shouldn't be placed on an incline to sleep and shouldn't be left unattended if they do fall asleep in a swing or stroller or car seat.

That doesn't mean not to use the gear. Car seats are a must when driving with a baby, and the AAP study points out that almost all car-seat-related deaths took place in a "nontraveling context," meaning outside the car. But the danger is real, if relatively rare. So be sure to use the devices as intended. And communicate the dangers to anyone else who takes care of your baby. The 2019 study found that, compared with other deaths, those in sitting devices were more likely to occur under the supervision of some sort of sitter or childcare provider than with the child's parents.

I know this is a scary subject. And I realize that there are plenty of times you can't imagine moving your sleeping baby and chancing waking him. But this is one more area where you want to be vigilant and observe safe sleep practices for your child.

On a Personal Note

WHEN OUR KIDS were little we frequently used the stroller or car seat to help them fall asleep. I remember repeating the same protocol numerous times with each child when they were babies. First, when my child closed his eyes, I'd perform that mental calculation—you know the one—to determine just how long to let him remain in the car seat before moving him to the crib. I had to give him time to get deep enough into his sleep that he wouldn't wake when I moved him, but not *so* long that if he did wake, he'd determine that he'd already had his nap and be up for the rest of the day. Any parent knows the pressure he or she can feel when aiming for that sweet spot.

Frequently I'd end up driving around the block multiple times to ensure I didn't create a radius so large that it would prevent me from making it home in time. I'd put on the familiar lullaby playlist to create the best sleepy environment and pray for the best. Far too often, though, my whole plan would be sabotaged when the baby's older brother, wide awake in his own car seat, would get fed up and end up yelling, "I'm so sick of these boring sleeping songs!" or "You just passed our house again! Why can't we go home?"

Smoking and Breastfeeding

You already know that smoking is harmful, for both you and your baby. But what if you're unable to give up the habit? Should you still breastfeed?

Competing Opinions

Perspective #1: Nicotine passes into breast milk, leading to many problems and preventing breastfeeding success while keeping your baby from sleeping well. If you can't quit smoking, at least avoid introducing this dangerous chemical into your infant's body.

Perspective #2: You should still nurse your baby, even if you smoke. He'll receive the advantages that come with nursing, which can counter some of the negative effects of your smoking.

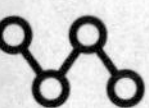

What the Science Says

EVEN THOUGH THEY'RE as aware as the rest of us about the harmful consequences, many breastfeeding women—as many as 7 percent to 16 percent—continue to smoke. Studies of the precise effects of postnatal nicotine exposure are limited, but recent reviews of the available literature offer a clear warning: Nicotine passes into breast milk and can negatively affect the breastfeeding process. And exposure to nicotine in breast milk has been associated with the possibility of negative effects on the baby, such as disturbed sleep patterns, liver and lung damage, and earlier weaning and shorter breastfeeding duration, which can affect infant cognition.

Aside from these direct health consequences, you want to remain mindful of the dangers of second- and thirdhand smoke. Research has established that exposure to secondhand smoke—plumes in the air—at any age can lead to lung cancer and heart disease. When children are exposed, it correlates with a higher risk of a variety of illnesses, including middle ear disease, breathing problems, and bacterial meningitis. It's also associated with colic and has been established as a cause of sudden infant death syndrome (SIDS). Thirdhand smoke is the residue left behind by smoking, which babies can access when they touch furniture and clothes near where the smoking has taken place.

As for the question of whether you should continue breastfeeding if you smoke, even though nicotine passes into breast milk, the answer is a resounding yes. The AAP and the CDC, along with numerous health experts, unequivocally state that breastfeeding still provides seemingly limitless benefits, even if the mother smokes. In fact, research shows that breastfeeding can even counteract some of the negative consequences your baby faces from your smoking.

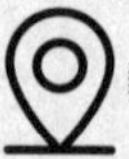

The Bottom Line

IF YOU CAN quit smoking, you should absolutely quit—for your health and your baby's. I know it's hard, but keep trying. If the best you can do is cut back, then cut back.

If you do continue smoking, take pains to avoid exposing your baby to second- and thirdhand smoke. You can do this by smoking soon after you've nursed (stretching out as much as possible the time between smoking and breastfeeding again) and by smoking outside instead of in the house or the car where your infant rides. Some experts recommend changing your clothes after smoking to decrease the amount of thirdhand smoke your infant will be exposed to. But yes, definitely keep breastfeeding, whether you're smoking or not. It's hard to overstate the advantages breast milk gives a child.

Social Media and Your Baby's Online Presence

In today's "digital-first" culture, is it OK to post pictures of your baby online? You want to share your joy, but what kind of concerns should you consider, particularly regarding safety and privacy?

Competing Opinions

Perspective #1: It's dangerous to let people access online photos of and information about your child. Even if you're in a closed group, you don't know what the others in the group will do with those pictures. Anyone can copy what you post and use it in any way they want. Plus, we should be careful about creating our children's original digital footprint when they don't have a say in what's being put into the world about them.

Perspective #2: We make plenty of decisions for our kids without waiting to hear what their preferences are. We're not undermining their right to privacy by letting Aunt Katinka see their Halloween costume. As for safety, sure, there are bad people in the world who will do bad things. But as long as you're wise about how much information you're sharing, avoiding giving specific details that someone could use to harm your child, there's nothing wrong with letting your friends and family join in the joy of watching as your baby grows and develops.

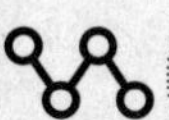

What the Science Says

"SHARENTING" IS A word that's been used to describe the practice of parents posting pictures of their kids online. While this phenomenon is being discussed and debated more and more widely, there's not a large body of research taking up the subject yet. General research is beginning to appear, with some of it focused specifically on babies. One conclusion we can draw with certainty is that sharenting has become the new normal. Even as far back as 2010, a survey found that more than 90 percent of two-year-olds and 80 percent of one-year-olds already had some form of an online presence.

One primary worry regarding this near-unanimous parenting phenomenon has to do with the safety of children. When a child's name, age, and location are available in a public forum like Facebook or Instagram, that child may be exposed to danger, either in the real world or in cyberspace. A recent problem is digital kidnapping, where a person steals images of a child and then uses them for their own purposes, sometimes claiming the child as their own or even sharing them on sites frequented by pedophiles.

The other key concern has to do with privacy. A baby won't have opinions on how you use her likeness on social media, but as she grows up, that will likely change. Some child advocates worry that by posting pictures of children, we take away some of their independence and autonomy. These people argue that a child ought to have the right to request that her parents not post a picture of her. And if an older child has that right, parents should be careful about making that decision without consideration for consequences and implications.

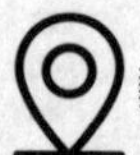

The Bottom Line

YOU'RE RIGHT TO wonder whether and when to post online photos and information about your child. Science is only beginning to explore the ramifications of this issue, and it doesn't offer much by way of guidance. There's no research that clearly argues against the practice, and parents are clearly willing to do so. But this is a frontier we've just begun to approach, and we'd be wise to keep our kids' safety and privacy in mind going forward.

Ultimately, you have to decide what you're comfortable with. It's true that as parents, we make all kinds of decisions for our children before they're old enough to weigh in and decide for themselves, and this is one of those areas where you can consider your own digital social circles, as well as your values, and make the decision that feels right to you.

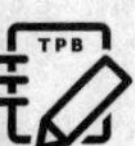

On a Personal Note

I POST PICTURES of my kids on social media, and I've done so since they were little. I've been careful to avoid offering too much identifying information, and I've tried to keep in mind how they might feel about certain shots once they're older. I've also typically chosen sites with settings that allowed me more control in terms of who was following me and who had access to my posts. But I haven't felt overly concerned about any negative consequences that might result from posting.

As my children have gotten older, we've had lots of ongoing conversations about digital presence. We have general guidelines in our family about posting information and pictures of one another, and these days I do ask their permission to post something that involves their picture or a story about them. (I ask the same courtesy of them, by the way, so I have the option to nix an unflattering photo or a picture I want to be kept private.)

I have a friend, though, who has made a point to avoid showing her children's faces in her social media. She still shares pictures of her experiences with her kids, but her daughter will typically be facing away from the camera as she rides the carousel, for example, or her son will be playing the piano with his eyes looking at the keyboard, preventing the viewer from seeing his face. I respect her caution and her awareness that those pictures are creating the beginnings of that child's digital footprint.

This issue, like so many having to do with technology and social media, is one that we'll all have to figure out along the way.

S

Spanking

Is spanking an effective and acceptable way to teach a baby lessons and deter unwanted behaviors?

Competing Opinions

Perspective #1: Spanking makes no sense—it doesn't work, and it's harmful. Babies' bodies and brains are too fragile, and children this age are developmentally unable to make the connection between spanking and a desired behavior. Plus, especially since parents of infants are by definition exhausted, there's greater potential for spanking to escalate into more serious harm. Babies need to trust their caregivers, and if their caregivers are inflicting pain on them, it can make the children feel unsafe in the world. There are simply more effective ways to discipline without the risks.

Perspective #2: It's definitely true that spanking in anger, or when the parent is out of control, should never take place. But spanking is a long-standing and trusted parental approach, and sometimes that's the only way babies can learn, especially if they're too young to understand logical explanations. So if a caregiver is calm and can spank in an intentional manner, it can be an effective way to teach a baby appropriate conduct and to discourage misbehavior.

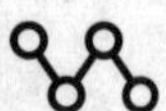

What the Science Says

I'LL FOCUS HERE on spanking in general, while highlighting information regarding the first year. Unless otherwise noted, I'm defining spanking the way it's described in current research literature, meaning corporal punishment where a parent uses an open palm and doesn't leave a mark.

I'm not, in other words, discussing harsh and frequent physical punishment. There's no debate in any of the literature that that type of discipline is ever effective or warranted. It does significant harm, impacting the developing brain in ways that can last a lifetime. (See the "Discipline" entry for more on an overall approach to discipline.)

As with most research, particularly in the social sciences, we can't claim proof with 100 percent certainty that all spanking of any kind leads to significantly negative outcomes for all children. While researchers have become increasingly methodical in how they control for variables that could skew their results, this is a difficult subject to study, especially when it comes to taking into account such varied contexts as culture, education, parental emotional state, researcher bias, how much conversation and explanation accompanies the discipline, how frequently it occurs, whether it's accompanied by affection and repair afterward, whether expectations have been communicated, and more.

Still, despite this caveat, we *can* say with great confidence that fifty years of research leans strongly in the direction of two general claims regarding spanking: (1) that it's ineffective in producing better long-term behavior, and (2) that it can lead to negative outcomes, many of them severe and significant.

Five key meta-analyses have appeared since 2002 looking at what the overall research says about spanking's effects on children. Each analysis acknowledges the difficulty of making claims of causality and other methodological challenges, but the overall conclusion we see again and again from reputable studies is that physical punishment is linked with negative child outcomes.

Each subsequent meta-analysis has improved on the earlier ones—for example, becoming more precise regarding the definition of "spanking"—and the evidence against spanking looks more and more compelling. Four of the five reviews come to decidedly confident conclusions regarding the correlations between spanking and negative outcomes. They point to individual studies determining that spanking is not effective as a long-term deterrent and linking it to various negative outcomes such as aggressive and difficult temperaments, defiance of parents, antisocial behavior, depression, anxiety, and hyperreactivity, to name only a few. In other words, according to these reviews, spanking may *increase* behavioral problems, not reduce them, and it can reduce overall well-being. The most recent and robust meta-analysis of available studies concludes by saying, "Parents who use spanking, practitioners who recommend it, and policymakers who allow it might reconsider doing so given that there is no evidence that spanking does any good for children and all evidence points to the risk of it doing harm."

One of the five meta-analyses disagrees, stopping short of determining that no benefits lead from spanking. It points to studies demonstrating specific examples when spanking can be effective to correct behavior. But even this review concludes by recommending that parents use "the mildest disciplinary response that will be effective for maintaining age-appropriate levels of cooperation" and points to a study finding that "the only use of spanking that has been demonstrated to be more effective than alternatives is when it is used to enforce time out when 2- to 6-year-olds refuse to comply with it." Its authors emphasize that what it calls "conditional spanking" should be "motivated by love" and used without anger and as a last resort "in such a way that reduces the need to use it in the future."

Two key observations about this outlying review should be highlighted. First, its focus is on whether or not spanking is "effective" for "reducing child compliance or antisocial behavior." Whereas many of the spanking opponents' arguments stress the negative effects on children's overall well-being, the attention here is on compliance. Also, regardless of their conclusions regarding the merits of occasional spanking, the authors of this review emphasize that it "should never be used in an infant's first 12 months of life."

Finally, it's worth noting that the AAP, the American Psychological Association, and the CDC have all reviewed the literature and issued formal policy statements against spanking and any form of corporal punishment. And as of 2018, more than fifty countries have banned physical punishment in schools and in homes.

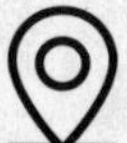

The Bottom Line

CERTAIN LIMITATIONS EXIST in the scientific literature on spanking, and more research is needed. That being said, though, the science that we do have overwhelmingly argues against spanking. More to the point of this book, even researchers who favor spanking in certain instances agree that it should never be used during the first year of a baby's life.

A Personal Note

I'M FIRMLY AGAINST spanking, for children of any age. In addition to the research studies, other bodies of literature in the child development and child-rearing sciences bolster opposition to spanking. Consider, for example, the neurobiological process that takes place during physical punishment. As mammals, we're wired to run to our parents when we're threatened in any way. But what if the parent is also the *source* of our pain and fear? Research exploring parent-child relationships has demonstrated over the last several decades that when a parent inflicts physical pain or produces significant fear within a child, that child faces an unresolvable biological paradox. One circuit drives the child *toward* their attachment figure for safety, while the other, competing circuit tries to escape the parent who's inflicting pain.

When we create this unresolvable biological paradox in our child's brain, it has the potential to produce all kinds of adverse long-term consequences. If we scare or inflict pain on our children, we activate the primitive-reactive brain, which then starts calling the shots, leading to *more* reactive behavior. Plus we risk teaching our kids that physical pain, used in the service of power and control, is the only alternative we could find to influence them—a lesson that can continue across the generations without some reflection.

Another primary reason I'm against spanking is that other options exist that not only are likely to be more effective but also can help build the problem-solving higher structures of the brain (instead of activating the reactive, lower mechanisms). Some parents begin their deliberation about how best to discipline by asking, "What punishment should I give in this instance?" That's actually the wrong question. Instead, we should ask, "What lesson do I want to teach here?" After all, that's what discipline is: teaching so that your child learns to be self-disciplined over time. If your child has misbehaved in some way, you of course want cooperation, to have her act in an appropriate manner. But you also want to teach her, helping her build skills so she can act more appropriately in the future. That's why you ask yourself, "What lesson do I want to teach here?" Some might believe that spanking is the best way to teach, but it activates a threat response in the nervous system, which means that little learning can take place. We have to be in a state where we are safe before we can learn. You can set clear limits and enforce boundaries—that's definitely important, and in a child's best interest—with your words and nonverbal communication, all while maintaining a nurturing connection with your child and helping her feel *safe*. Doing so will give you a much better chance of achieving your goal of building skills that will lead to better behavior and a more fully developed conscience down the road. It tends to strengthen your relationship with your child as well.

In other words, rather than immediately offering punishment, it's often more effective to connect emotionally with a child, engaging the higher, more sophisticated, thinking parts of her brain. By relying on respectful conversation and connection, we can (and should) still set limits, but in a caring manner. Then our children can learn to make healthy and thoughtful choices while handling their emotions well, all while understanding that they can come to us, share their mistakes, and be safe.

My final point is a caution: spanking can escalate into greater violence. Every parent—and for sure anyone who's ever taken care of an infant while working on a far-too-limited amount of sleep—knows that anger and frustration can rise to the surface when we least expect it. We can lose control *so* easily. One minute you're changing a diaper while your infant squirms and resists; then you find yourself holding him down; then, in your sleep-deprived state, all of a sudden you feel the urge to swat him or shake him. This kind of reaction can happen to anyone.

The problem with allowing even the possibility of spanking your child "under certain circumstances" is that you're setting up a terrible risk of doing something more extreme in a moment of weakness or rage than you ever intended. And the fragility of a baby means that shaking, twisting, shoving, and so on can lead to tragic results. Studies have found that children spanked at age one are 33 percent more likely to be involved in a child protective services issue than non-spanked babies, and spanked babies are more likely to be abused and to sustain a physical injury.

Deciding not to spank won't prevent you from losing control and acting in ways you know you shouldn't. But if you begin from the position that you're never going to inflict *any* kind of physical harm at all on your baby, you're at least starting that much farther away from that scary endpoint.

For all of these reasons, I strongly oppose spanking. I believe that all children should feel safe, to not be hit or hurt by their caregivers. I believe the research will continue to prove more emphatically the negative effects of spanking, and that eventually we will reach a tipping point, where children who are spanked are in the minority.

I also know that some of you reading this will regret that you've spanked your child in the past. Be gracious with yourself and recognize that you were doing your best with what you knew then, and now you know more. It's not too late to make a change. Children benefit hugely when we make positive changes, so commit now to always choosing safety and connection while you set boundaries.

Spoiling a Baby by Too Much Holding

New parents often receive conflicting advice about holding their baby, and what messages they're sending when they respond to every cry. Is it possible to "spoil" an infant by giving her too much attention?

Competing Opinions

Perspective #1: Frequently holding your baby or responding every time she cries will make her spoiled and teach her that she can manipulate you into responding whenever she wants you nearby. Of course you're going to hold your infant a lot, but don't feel as if you have to respond every time she asks. It's important that kids learn to soothe themselves, so that they don't grow up too dependent or entitled.

Perspective #2: Babies are cognitively incapable of manipulation, and you can't spoil them through affection, holding them too much, or responding to their cries. Of course you have to take care of your own needs, but hold your baby as much as you can and as much as she needs. That'll strengthen the relationship and create trust between the two of you. And doing so comes with numerous health and developmental benefits.

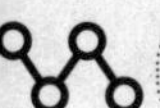

What the Science Says

RESEARCH HAS CLEARLY shown the benefits of skin-to-skin contact with newborns. Sometimes known as "kangaroo care," this practice was developed in Colombia by Dr. Nathalie Charpak in the 1970s to help low-birth-weight infants, since the prevailing treatment had been to keep them in incubators with little human interaction. Since then, the practice of skin-to-skin contact has become routine in hospital nurseries. Its benefits for newborns, and particularly preterm, low-birth-weight infants, have been verified in numerous studies.

Longitudinal research over many decades has demonstrated that when parents respond quickly and sensitively to their child's cries, it does not make the child more dependent but rather promotes independence because the child comes to trust that the caregiver will be there when needed and keep them safe when a need is communicated.

Especially when there's skin-to-skin contact, holding a baby produces a list of benefits—for both parent and child—that goes on and on. It promotes social development, encourages the growth of the social aspects of the brain, and has been shown to reduce pain during certain medical procedures. It results in lower stress levels, better-regulated body temperatures, and an increase in relational trust. It increases success in breastfeeding and has been shown to reduce crying and increase contentment among newborns.

Particularly for premature babies or infants who have had difficult or even traumatic births, skin-to-skin contact and gentle, nurturing touch have been shown to result in long-lasting benefits like enhanced brain development, higher IQ, lower rates of aggression and behavioral problems, and less hyperactivity and absenteeism in school.

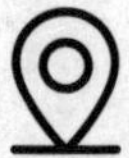

The Bottom Line

STUDIES HAVE CONSISTENTLY shown that not only is holding babies early and often not going to harm them; it's essential and has long-term positive impacts on their health and development. Physical touch is critical to your child's optimal development and health. You cannot hold, touch, pick up, or love your baby too much. Tremendous health, emotional, relational, and developmental benefits come from spending as much time physically connected to your baby as you enjoy and as your baby needs.

As for the message you're sending when you respond to your infant's cries? Yes, he's going to learn the lesson that when he needs you, you'll be there for him. What better message do you want to send repeatedly at this early stage? You won't be creating dependence or selfishness. Research shows that this kind of consistent response to his emotional needs actually creates an attachment that will make him feel confident and *more* independent as he grows up. He will be more willing to take healthy risks and face life's challenges with resilience. (See the entry "Discipline.")

That goes not just for newborns but for older babies as well. Even as your infant approaches and passes one year, he'll still want and need to be held. He'll be fussy from time to time, and you won't always want to hold him. But as long as you can do it, be there for him (as much as your back can handle). Yes, of course, you have to practice self-care and find time to be away from your baby for the sake of your own sanity and well-being. But when you two are together, don't ever wonder whether you are somehow doing harm by picking him up when he needs you. I'll repeat: you cannot hold, touch, pick up, or love your baby too much.

Stranger Anxiety

Stranger anxiety, also known as infant shyness, represents a normal stage in the life of an infant. It will likely be most intense around seven to ten months of age, coinciding with the baby having become more attached to you and the members of her immediate family. Your infant's discomfort around strangers might be only a short phase or it could last a good bit longer. For most kids it passes within a year or two.

How can you avoid pushing your baby too hard into new situations, while still helping her become comfortable around strangers as well as the new faces she'll encounter as her social world expands? Is allowing a stranger to hold your infant a beneficial step in the process of socialization? Or should you be more protective?

Competing Opinions

Perspective #1: Protect your baby, of course, and when she shows signs of feeling stressed or overwhelmed, you obviously need to pull back and give her time to regulate and regain her calm. But it's good for her to be introduced to new people and to see that she can get through and deal with moments where she's uncomfortable. Interactions with others will help her build confidence and social skills from infancy.

Perspective #2: Aware that your baby's fear is a natural stage of development, you should be careful about pushing her to interact with new people before she's ready. Responding to her cues and natural inclinations is part of respecting her and helping her build trust. She'll have plenty of time down the road to develop social skills; when she's this young, it's important to help her feel safe and to let her know that you're there for her and will keep her safe, both physically and emotionally.

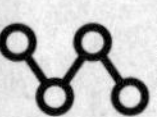

What the Science Says

THE KEY FINDING to keep in mind is that stranger anxiety is a perfectly typical stage in a child's development. Studies have demonstrated this primary fact for decades, so there's nothing to worry about if your baby suddenly leans away when she meets Uncle Dave for the first time. Aside from this, we can point to certain findings that can guide us as we nurture our children through whatever fear or anxiety they're encountering when they meet new people.

For example, research shows that how a parent responds when encountering a stranger influences a baby's reaction. In one study, mothers were taught how to display non-anxious mannerisms as well as socially anxious behaviors, and to exhibit those tendencies when meeting new people with their infants. As expected, the babies of the mothers who appeared nervous and uncomfortable "were significantly more fearful and avoidant with the stranger" themselves.

Other interesting work has been done on infants' ability to distinguish strangers from non-strangers by the sound of their laughter. Even as young as five months, babies can learn to glean important information from specific acoustic characteristics of laughter, then "index" that data in such a way that allows them to determine the social relationship—whether the new person is a friend or a stranger. As the authors of the study put it, "Infants heard co-laughter between friends and co-laughter between strangers [as] depicting one of two different social contexts: either two people affiliating or turning away from each other." Once again, the babies were reading their parents' cues and responding accordingly.

One other dynamic that's important to consider is the importance of temperament. Research clearly demonstrates the importance of parents adjusting their expectations and approaches depending on their child's personality and temperament. A baby who feels more shy or sensitive is going to respond to one parental behavior and not another, whereas a more outgoing child could behave completely differently. (See "Sensitive Babies.")

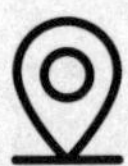

The Bottom Line

NOT ONLY DO babies follow their parents' cues when it comes to social interactions with people they don't know, but they can also be very perceptive to subtle nuances within relationships. Add the fact that temperament can lead one child to be comfortable being held by a stranger at the grocery store and another one to be wary even around Grandma, and it's no wonder there are questions about how best to respond to a baby's stranger anxiety.

Where does all this lead us? As with so many other parenting questions, it all comes back to relationship. You want to get to know your child—your unique, individual child—well enough that you can recognize the moments when she needs to bury her face in your chest and be allowed to stay there, as opposed to the situations when, with a bit of encouragement, she might be willing to come out of her shell a little. Based on the intimacy of your relationship and mutual understanding, you can find a way to thread the needle and avoid the two extremes. You don't want to push her so hard that she ends up becoming even more reluctant to socialize the next time she meets a stranger. But you also want to give her opportunities to understand that she can handle a certain amount of discomfort, and that it can be fun to meet new people and try new experiences.

One other point: As parents, we can too quickly move to compare our child with others' and assume that there's a "normal" way children should behave. When it comes to personality and temperament, this parental tendency can be especially problematic. Yes, your sister's baby might smile and laugh for new people he meets, and your baby might be more naturally withdrawn and reticent about warming up to others. In that case, you need to show up for your child and support her with whatever she needs, not push her to act in ways that simply aren't who she is at that time.

Helping your infant to be comfortable around people outside her family, to cope with the stranger anxiety that's often a natural part of her social development, takes your patience and presence. If your baby is uncomfortable with strangers, or even with members of your extended family who want to hold her, there's no need to rush. Ask them to wait a bit for her to feel more secure. Introduce her to new people, but stay close—your presence will reassure her, and her ability to tolerate new people and experiences will expand over time.

S

Sunscreen

You know the importance of protecting your baby from the sun's damage. Should sunscreen be one of your protective measures? Are there any risks that outweigh the benefit of guarding against ultraviolet radiation (UVR)?

Competing Opinions

Perspective #1: Sunscreen is a must for babies. The best thing is to keep them in the shade because of their delicate skin, but sun exposure is going to take place practically anytime you're outside, so use sunscreen for an added layer of protection.

Perspective #2: Avoid sunscreen whenever you can. Its chemicals can irritate the skin and cause other unintended side effects. Instead, keep your baby covered up and in the shade.

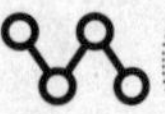

What the Science Says

THE KEY POINT here is one you already know: sun can damage skin and lead to significant problems, the most notable being skin cancer. And you likely also know that infants' skin is especially vulnerable to the sun's effects, since it is immature and an inadequate barrier against hazardous agents such as UVR. The earlier in life that the DNA is exposed to UVR, the greater the damage that can take place. Experts therefore stress the importance of protecting children's skin.

Sunscreen, though, is not the automatic answer, at least for the first six months of a baby's life. The problem is that because of their low body mass, they have an increased potential for absorbing chemicals into their skin, and their metabolic systems won't be able to detoxify the chemicals.

(That applies to all infants, regardless of complexion, race, or ethnic background.) Because of this danger, organizations including the AAP, the CDC, and the American Academy of Dermatology all recommend against using sunscreen until a child is at least six months old.

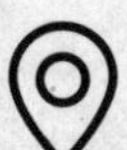

The Bottom Line

THE FIRST RULE if you're going to be in the sun is to protect your child. Ideally, that will mean having her in a hat and clothes that cover her skin, and still keeping her in the shade. That's a good rule of thumb to keep in mind throughout her childhood, by the way, especially if her complexion is fair. Just remember that the younger she is, the more damage sun can do.

For the first six months you may not find it that challenging to keep her in the shade. As she begins to move, crawl, and eventually walk, though, it will become more and more difficult. At that time you should absolutely use sunscreen (while still minimizing the time she spends in direct sunlight whenever possible). Just do your homework about which sunscreens are healthiest for young children, and watch for any adverse reactions you may need to discuss with your pediatrician.

S

Swaddling

Swaddling, or wrapping a baby's body in a thin blanket or sheet, has been practiced for centuries. Many modern parents love it and say it promotes both sleep and security for the baby, but some fear that it may not be safe and could even lead to suffocation, sudden infant death syndrome (SIDS), or some other form of sudden unexpected infant death (SUID).

Competing Opinions

Perspective #1: Swaddling calms infants when they're upset, and it promotes sleep by re-creating the security and snugness of the womb. Swaddled babies spontaneously wake up less often and cry less than those who aren't swaddled.

Perspective #2: The risks associated with swaddling outweigh any benefits. SIDS isn't the only danger. Swaddling can also lead to overheating, and it can affect a baby's physical development and even cause hip dysplasia.

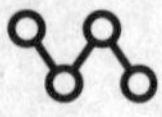

What the Science Says

WHILE THERE'S NOT a conclusive body of research, the science seems to point to the fact that swaddling presents minimal risk if precautions are taken and it's done the right way. Certain hazards do exist. For example, swaddling too tightly around the hips seems correlated with the possibility of hip dysplasia, though it's not clear whether such swaddling actually causes the dysplasia or simply worsens the condition in infants already predisposed to it. But this problem appears to be avoided when you use a safe, "hip-healthy" technique, where the swaddling is loose around the hips.

As for SIDS, a 2016 meta-analysis and a 2017 integrative review both found that, while consistent and conclusive research studies were limited, there didn't appear to be a clear association between swaddling and SIDS. Instead, the link existed more clearly between SIDS and unsafe swaddling techniques, like using thick sheets or blankets that could lead to overheating, or placing a baby on his front or side rather than laying him on his back.

Research does support the claims of swaddling proponents, finding that babies wrapped securely have greater "sleep efficiency." They are less likely to wake themselves as a result of hypnagogic startles, the involuntary reflex that results in a sudden body jerk. Swaddling has been found to be soothing when an infant is overstimulated, and it can help him cry less often.

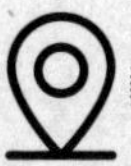

The Bottom Line

THIS IS ONE of those decisions that's entirely up to you. If you decide to swaddle, having understood the risks and benefits, be sure to read guidelines for safe and effective swaddling. These will likely involve placing your baby on his back, watching out for overheating, wrapping him securely so he can't unwrap himself (but not so tight that his legs and feet can't move freely), and making sure to stop swaddling as soon as he shows signs of rolling over on his own. A quick online search will lead you to more specifics about the dos and don'ts of swaddling.

S

Swimming

Swimming lessons for infants and toddlers continue to gain in popularity. Should you sign your baby up?

Competing Opinions

Perspective #1: No preschooler is ever "water-safe," but teaching your infant to swim may prevent drowning in case he accidentally falls into the pool. Not only that, there's some evidence that lessons are beneficial for physical growth, balance, and coordination. At the very least, infant aquatic programs can introduce babies to the joy of being in the water.

Perspective #2: Swimming lessons don't reduce the risk of drowning for infants, and it's dangerous to make that claim. Other considerable risks are involved because babies are still so fragile. Getting babies comfortable with going into water before they have the ability to be fully water-safe gives them a false sense of confidence, increasing the danger. In a few years, once their motor skills are further developed, swimming lessons will be a must. But at this age, kids aren't ready.

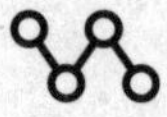

What the Science Says

ON THE PLUS side, there are studies showing that babies who learn to swim experience physical benefits and outperform their peers for several years on various skills like balance and grasping objects. Another study shows both cognitive and physical advances for babies who swim, but this particular study is methodologically flawed since it was sponsored by the swimming-school industry and relied on parental reporting rather than observed performance.

In addition, authorities such as the AAP encourage swimming lessons for children from one to four years old and acknowledge that lessons can help reduce drowning risk. For kids younger than one, the AAP endorses parent-child water-play classes as a fun way for parent and child to interact while getting the infant used to being in the pool.

However, when it comes to expecting babies to actually swim, authorities express more warnings than endorsements. Swimming is associated with dangers other than drowning—for example, ear concerns, water intoxication (swallowing too much water), and various infectious diseases—and infants can be especially at risk due to their young age and immature development. Because of babies' delicate immune systems, some doctors recommend keeping babies under six months out of lakes and chlorinated pools.

Beyond that, though, kids in general simply aren't developmentally ready for actual swimming until they're at least four, and for many kids proper motor development acquisition won't happen until closer to five, when children aren't "limited by their neuromuscular capacity." Yes, babies under one may show reflexive swimming movements, but they're not old enough to hold their heads out of the water well enough to breathe and keep themselves safe.

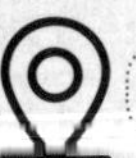

The Bottom Line

ENJOYING SWIM TIME with your baby can be a fun and safe experience for both of you. It may even allow your baby to be less apprehensive when he's older and ready for swimming lessons. But for the time being, it's best and safest not to rely on any company's claims that they can teach your infant to swim, much less be pool-safe.

None of this means you can't participate with your baby in aquatic instruction and have fun introducing him to the idea of swimming. But authorities are simply going to be very cautious anytime we're talking about water. Tragedy can occur in so many ways when it comes to children, and especially an infant. Be particularly watchful.

Whatever you decide regarding swimming lessons and water safety, avoid becoming overconfident. Even if your little one develops the ability to go underwater and swim back to the surface, by no means should that make you comfortable taking your eyes off of him anytime he's in the water. As he grows over the next couple of years and becomes more self-assured in the water, the same warning applies. Tragedy can strike in an instant, and lessons providing some amount of water competence for infants and toddlers should never be considered a fail-safe way to avoid the risk of drowning. This holds true with infants, toddlers, and young children around any body of water, including bathtubs, buckets of water, fountains, and so on. Toddlers' heads are heavy in comparison to their bodies, and should they fall headfirst into water, even in a bucket, they may not be able to pull their heads out of it.

On a Personal Note

MANY BABIES LOVE water. But more than a few times I've been asked for advice from new parents who had negative experiences when they tried to get their babies comfortable with swimming. Typically, they signed up for parent-baby classes and found that their babies *hated* being in the pool. Rather than reinforcing the fun and idyllic image in their minds, the class became torture. Their swimming instructors often emphasized the importance of sticking with it to get the babies used to the water, but the parents' instincts told them it didn't feel right.

I often teach that while intermittent tolerable stress with enough support and care can be good for our children in order to build resilience, the brain makes neural associations between emotional/physiological states and our experiences. So while water safety is essential by a certain age, it doesn't have to come during infanthood. Swimming lessons can even prove counterproductive, creating negative associations with getting in the pool, which may result in more obstacles to overcome when it's time to learn to swim.

Make water play fun and safe for your baby so that he can have positive associations with learning to swim. But there's no rush right now. If it makes him miserable, just take a break and try again in a few months.

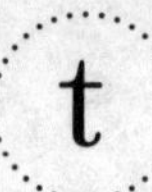

Teaching Babies to "Read"

In today's achievement-oriented society, many parents want to give their infants a head start in learning the skills they'll need to succeed in school and beyond. Books, apps, flash cards, media, and other learning tools are marketed to parents of children as young as three months old. Does direct instruction, particularly in reading skills, work for infants? Will it turn your child into a "Baby Einstein"?

Competing Opinions

Perspective #1: You should definitely be reading to your baby, but there's no reason to begin the "grill and drill" process at this age. Let babies be babies. They'll learn by simply interacting with the world, playing, and living their day-to-day lives. There will be more than enough time for formal instruction later.

Perspective #2: *Sesame Street* has been proven to help preschoolers be more prepared for kindergarten, so why not go a step further and begin teaching reading earlier? Helping your baby succeed should be one of your biggest priorities as a parent, and you have a responsibility to push your child to reach his full potential. There are many options for programs and learning tools for babies, and while maybe you can't say for sure that they'll improve your child's reading comprehension in a few years, how can it hurt to provide some early instruction, whether or not it gives him an edge academically? Plus, aside from exercising your child's brain, reading together is a nice bonding experience for the two of you.

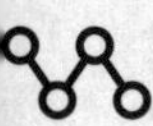

What the Science Says

OVER THE LAST couple of decades, numerous studies have examined whether popular "teach your baby to read" programs actually deliver on what they promise. Most of these investigations have found that babies are incapable of learning to read, despite parents claiming that their babies have indeed learned to recognize words.

Much of the debate appears to come down to the definition of the word "read." I won't go into the minutiae of the argument, but to simplify a bit, investigators define reading as comprehension of the relationships among the letters, the words, and the concepts or objects they represent. Researchers draw a distinction between actually *reading* and what many parents are observing, where their infant can look at a word—for example, "gorilla"—and then point to a picture of a primate (even though they can't even pronounce the word yet). Two different studies have attempted to clarify the researchers' point by demonstrating that children as young as two and a half could accurately identify logos and familiar images—like a McDonald's billboard or a stop sign—but that they were unable to recognize the same words without the familiar context. Thus, the toddlers weren't technically reading as much as identifying an image in context.

The research examining screen-centric approaches to teaching very young children to read is especially damning. For one thing, too much screen time has the potential to negatively affect children cognitively, relationally, and physically. Links have been found between television viewing and problems such as diminished executive function (critical thinking, self-control, focus, decision-making, etc.), weaker theory-of-mind skills (social-cognitive abilities that allow us to consider and understand the mental states of ourselves and others), and obesity. While the studies offering these findings looked at older kids, not babies, and focused exclusively on television viewing, as opposed to a broader view of screen time, they still suggest potential negative outcomes from too much viewing time. (See the entry "Screen Time" for more details about navigating the benefits and perils that accompany the ubiquity of screens in our lives.)

As for learning to read, there's practically no persuasive evidence that babies, especially during the first year, are going to acquire anything of value in terms of preparedness for formal education by looking at a screen. Obviously, babies begin building the basics of language and vocabulary very early—the evidence could not be more clear on the importance of talking and reading with even the youngest of children, and that evidence continues to grow. But research compellingly shows that linguistic and cognitive development, obviously essential for reading, occurs at this age *in relationship*—interacting with live persons, not with a video on a screen. In fact, one study that does find that infants and toddlers can learn from screen media argues that this learning occurs only under the right circumstances: when the child has certain capabilities, the quality of the video content is high, and the process is relational (that is, the child receives the involvement and attention of a parent or other co-viewer).

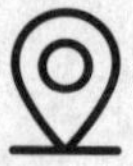

The Bottom Line

IF YOU WANT to give your baby a head start in learning all the things he needs to succeed in his future, the best place to start is with you. Your baby was born to learn, and you can help by talking to him, reading and singing to him, counting his fingers and toes, and allowing him to safely explore his world.

It's virtually impossible to overemphasize the importance of reading *to* your baby. As for teaching your infant to read, there doesn't seem to be any evidence demonstrating that children this young can be taught to actually read, as it's defined by experts. That being said, while critics have argued that infancy reading programs are a waste of time and money, no research exists showing that the programs are producing detrimental effects.

So here's the bottom line: There's no science-based reason to invest time and money in programs that promise to teach your baby to read. If you want to do it, you're likely doing no harm. In fact, as long as you're not attached to academic benefits or outcomes, if you enjoy spending time with your baby this way and your baby enjoys it, go for it. But it's certainly not necessary, and there are plenty of other ways you can introduce him to the fun and magic of language, simply by spending time and interacting with him. His world is his classroom, and you—your voice, your attention, and your presence—are his best teacher.

Teething Necklaces

Amber teething necklaces have become popular with parents over the last decade, with proponents arguing that wearing the necklaces will release a substance—succinic acid—into the infant's skin and ease the discomfort of teething. Does it actually work? Should you give it a shot?

Competing Opinions

Perspective #1: Any claim that wearing an amber necklace will relieve teething pain simply by lying against a baby's skin is nothing more than pseudoscience.

Perspective #2: It might sound crazy, but parents who have tried out the necklaces have found that their infants experience less teething pain and experience longer periods of calm.

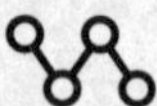

What the Science Says

THIS IS ONE of those subjects where there's not much ambiguity. Avoid the amber teething necklaces.

For one thing, there's no science that actually supports that they work, and the supposed science that proponents point to in support of amber beads' analgesic qualities has been shown to be false. Beyond that, authorities are virtually unanimous that the necklaces present a significant suffocation hazard because a baby might swallow the beads and choke, and there's a risk of strangulation because the clasp of the necklace might not easily release.

As a result, organizations such as the AAP, the Canadian Paediatric Society, and the FDA have warned parents not to use teething jewelry such as amber necklaces.

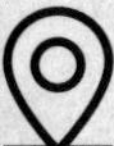

The Bottom Line

WHILE SOME PARENTS swear by them, amber teething necklaces (along with any other type of necklace) should be avoided for babies. I know you don't like seeing your little one suffer, but there are better ways to offer relief. Find alternatives, like rubbing your child's gums with a clean finger or offering something safe to chew on, like a cool, wet facecloth or a teething ring made of firm rubber.

t

Teething Numbing Gels

Your baby is teething and in pain. Is it OK to use one of the numbing gels on the market?

Competing Opinions

Perspective #1: There are decent-sized problems with the gels you can buy at the pharmacy. Avoid them and stick to the traditional teething products and remedies.

Perspective #2: Teething gels are just another tool in your toolbox in caring for your infant. If there's a method for providing relief from pain, use it.

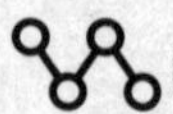

What the Science Says

LOCAL ANESTHETICS, LIKE over-the-counter gum-numbing gels containing benzocaine, should definitely be avoided when treating a teething infant. The same goes for prescribed medicine containing viscous lidocaine, a drug used for adults with sores in their mouth. Some parents dip pacifiers into lidocaine to address a child's teething pain. In a word, don't.

The American Academy of Pediatrics and the American Academy of Pediatric Dentists both caution against teething gels. And in warnings regarding homeopathic teething tablets and gels, the FDA explains that these products often haven't been evaluated or approved for safety or efficacy and can lead to medical problems including constipation, agitation, and seizures. Numerous studies support these warnings, finding that topical benzocaine can lead to other significant adverse health effects including brain injury and heart problems. The FDA also makes its strongest warning against treating infant teething pain using medicines containing viscous lidocaine, cautioning that doing so could result in serious harm and even death.

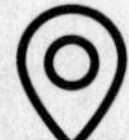

The Bottom Line

HERE'S ANOTHER CASE of the importance of sticking with the tried and true. As the previous section recommended, a cool wet cloth is a great thing to give your teething baby. So is a hard rubber teething ring. Or you can rub your clean finger on the gums. But completely avoid teething gels along with those amber-bead necklaces (see "Teething Necklaces").

t

Thumb Sucking

Even when we understand that thumb sucking is a natural, calming activity for our infant, we can feel uncomfortable if the habit persists. The question is, how long is too long? At what age might thumb sucking result in damage to your baby's permanent teeth or teasing at daycare?

Competing Opinions

Perspective #1: Thumb sucking is a natural behavior in infants that can be a way of self-soothing. Most babies will give it up on their own soon enough, so this is one of those things you can relax about.

Perspective #2: It's not the world's worst problem, but prolonged thumb sucking may lead to your child being teased, and if it lasts long enough it can have a damaging effect on speech and incoming teeth. You never know how long it will last, so it's best to nip it in the bud.

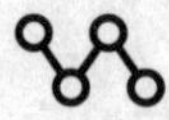

What the Science Says

THE CONSISTENT MESSAGE from both research and pediatric authorities is that thumb sucking is perfectly typical and nothing to worry about. Babies are born with the need to suck; many start sucking their thumbs in the womb. So there's no cause for concern for the first couple of years of your child's life. After that, various studies have found complications appearing after three to five years, depending on which study you look at.

The primary negative outcomes relate to oral issues. Dental problems can occur if the child is still sucking her thumb once her permanent teeth begin to come in. It's not only the alignment of teeth that can be affected but the roof of the mouth as well, so at some point a pediatric dentist might recommend a mouth "appliance" as a deterrent to sucking. Also, one study has found that if kids suck their fingers or use a pacifier past the age of three, they're more likely to develop speech impediments.

The news isn't all bad, though. At one point it was assumed that thumb sucking was evidence of insecurity and/or anxiety in children. Now, though, most researchers see it as simply learned behavior that's neither a cause nor a symptom of insecurity or some sort of psychological problem. There's even some evidence of beneficial effects. One study concluded that allergies may be reduced in children who bite their nails and suck their thumbs. The researchers make a point to note, in case you're wondering, that they do not recommend trying to get kids to take up these habits.

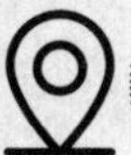

The Bottom Line

IT'S NOT PROBLEMATIC or uncommon for your baby to suck her thumb. In fact, it's quite natural as a tool she can use to self-soothe. In all likelihood, she'll wean herself from her thumb on her own. But if she doesn't, there's little need to be concerned unless she chooses to persist after her permanent teeth begin to come in. Then some positive encouragement and gentle reassurance from you, along with the likely peer pressure she'll receive from other kids, can help her break the habit.

t

Tummy Time

For the last couple of decades or so, pediatricians have been recommending a few minutes of supervised tummy time, or front-down play, to help babies strengthen their necks and arms so they can progress toward what are known as "prone skills," such as rolling over, pushing up, and eventually crawling. But some question the necessity of tummy time. How important is it for your infant's healthy development?

Competing Opinions

Perspective #1: Tummy time strengthens babies' neck, arm, and shoulder muscles and improves their motor skills so they can move toward learning to crawl and eventually walk. It gives them a breather from being on their backs, helping prevent flat spots on their head. Plus it can be fun to be joined on the floor by Mom or Dad, who might bring along a toy or other fun object.

Perspective #2: If babies can roll onto their stomachs on their own, it makes sense to give them the chance to push themselves up and look around in that position. But until they can do it independently, tummy time is going to make them unhappy and even confused, since they're not strong enough to hold up their heads and comfortably see what's going on around them. We should honor their natural development and allow them to move to new milestone moments when they're ready.

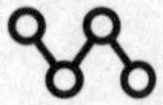

What the Science Says

A FEW YEARS after pediatricians started recommending that babies be placed on their backs to sleep in order to reduce the risk of sudden infant death syndrome (SIDS), researchers began to notice that back sleeping appeared to be resulting in two negative consequences: the development of plagiocephaly (a flattening of the back or side of the head) and delayed rolling over and crawling due to reduced muscle tone. Tummy time was introduced to address these concerns, and pediatricians have been recommending it for years now.

Opponents of tummy time point to the effects it can have on a baby's emotional state, since infants often feel uncomfortable in the prone position. One study noted that infants who hadn't been exposed to consistent periods of tummy time were especially likely to cry and even become distressed when placed in the position. Others argue that tummy time isn't necessary and is an overreaction by authorities claiming causal outcomes when none exists. Their argument is that the recommendation resulted from fears that babies were spending too much time on their backs. But these critics point out that even when this is true, babies are also being held or sitting in carriers and strollers for plenty of time throughout the day, meaning they're not always supine.

Still, both the AAP and the NIH definitively recommend supervised tummy time for babies, beginning virtually as soon as they are born. As the AAP puts it, "Back to sleep, tummy to play."

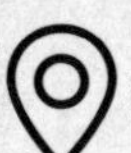

The Bottom Line

THE SCIENCE is very clear when it comes to sleeping position: babies should be placed on their backs to reduce the risk of SIDS. Then, according to the experts, when they wake, supervised tummy time really is a good idea. Two or three minutes is plenty of time early on; then your baby will be able to handle more along the way. Tummy time should definitely *not* lead to distress. Some frustration is OK, as long as your child also feels loved, supported, and connected to you in the process. You can even place her prone on your chest instead of the floor—whatever makes it palatable. Then along the way, it can give the two of you a little face time

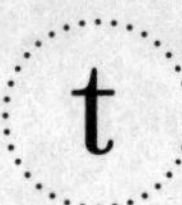

where you're both on the floor enjoying each other. For variety, add toys or involve an older sibling in the fun.

On a Personal Note

I WANTED TO do what all the books said to give my firstborn every advantage, so soon after we got home from the hospital, I put him on a cute blanket for tummy time. He would just lie there, facedown or with his head to the side, and cry. I tried to comfort him for a minute, then I shrugged, picked him up, and decided to try later when he could better tolerate it and begin to enjoy it. Over time, he did.

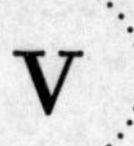

Vaccinations

What does the latest research say about vaccines, and should you follow the guidelines set by organizations such as the CDC and the AAP? How seriously should you take the claims that some of the vaccines produce dangerous side effects?

Competing Opinions

Perspective #1: Vaccines contain harmful ingredients that can have dangerous side effects, including an increased risk of autism. The government shouldn't have the power to dictate questionable health requirements to parents. In fact, some of the illnesses targeted by the vaccines—like chicken pox, measles, and rubella—are relatively harmless and can be treated with common household products and home remedies. So why inject potentially dangerous drugs into your child? Rather than relying on vaccination, you're much better off counting on his natural, innate immune system.

Perspective #2: Vaccines can save your baby's life and the lives of others, and they've helped us eradicate life-threatening diseases. They're safe according to major medical and health organizations, and the FDA requires years and years of testing before vaccines can be licensed. Negative health reactions to immunizations are rare, and by preventing illness, they also save parents time and money.

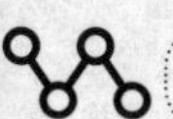

What the Science Says

LET'S START WITH an abbreviated list of world medical organizations stating that vaccines are safe: the WHO, the AAP, the CDC, the American Academy of Family Physicians, the United Nations Foundation, the FDA, the American Medical Association, the U.S. Department of Health and Human Services, the Canadian Paediatric Society, and the National Foundation for Infectious Diseases.

Most people are going to find this list pretty compelling. It's not that health organizations can't be wrong, manipulated, or compromised in some way by money or politics or other forces. But for parents to choose not to vaccinate their children, they have to make that decision going against a great deal of medical momentum from the leading health organizations.

But what are these organizations basing their recommendations on? One factor would be the number of illnesses prevented via vaccines. Without going into all the minutiae of the available data, we can look at various numbers that point to wide-ranging benefits associated with vaccinations—specifically, in terms of preventing children's deaths.

There's data, for example, on lives saved and diseases avoided by childhood immunization. According to the CDC, since 1994, vaccinations have prevented an estimated 419 million illnesses, 26.8 million hospitalizations, and 936,000 early deaths of children. We can also look at lives that *could be* saved by vaccinations but aren't. UNICEF reports that each year, 453,000 children die from rotavirus, 476,000 from pneumococcus, 199,000 from *Haemophilus influenzae* type b (Hib), 195,000 from pertussis, 118,000 from the measles, and 60,000 from tetanus. Each of these 1.5 million deaths were from diseases that were preventable via vaccines, highlighting both the benefits of immunization and the ultimate cost of its absence.

The benefits of vaccines can be generational as well. Women who have been immunized against measles, mumps, and rubella (MMR) have greatly decreased chances of passing on the illnesses to their babies and thereby avoiding the birth defects that can come with them. Add to that the fact that some diseases, such as smallpox, no longer even exist, and we can see that immunizations can offer health not only in the present but in the future as well.

But are vaccines actually safe? In other words, scientific authorities are clearly affirming the efficacy of immunizations. But what are the risks? Specifically, what are the risks for your child? Let's handle the big one first. There's no evidence that vaccines cause autism. In fact, the original study that initiated the debate years ago has since been not only forcefully debunked but retracted.

But autism is not the only concern that makes some parents wary about vaccinations. There are other risks that are more credible, according to research. As the CDC acknowledges, all vaccines come with a risk of side effects, ranging from mild local reactions (which are the most frequent) to severe allergic reactions such as anaphylaxis (which are very rare). Research points to other adverse effects as well, some of which can be minor—fussiness, a low-grade fever, fatigue, soreness, and so on—while some are more significant, such as fainting or a febrile seizure associated with a high fever.

However, scientific analyses of the available research consistently contextualize the danger, pointing out not only the benefits that are much more likely—the AAP asserts that "most childhood vaccines are 90 percent–99 percent effective in preventing disease"—but also the extreme rarity of the most concerning risks. If a child isn't vaccinated and is immunocompromised, then additional threats can obviously crop up, as can the likelihood of dangerous outcomes, possibly even death in extreme cases. (One study found that an unexpected consequence of unvaccinated children is that several acquired measles while waiting in their pediatricians' offices for other matters.) But research shows that negative consequences from immunization, in contrast, are so rare that, especially compared to the benefits provided, they're simply not worth worrying about.

Some parents wonder about an alternative or delayed vaccination schedule, where immunizations are spread out over a longer time period so that babies don't receive so many vaccines at once. One practical downside is that by drawing out the timetable, babies end up having to get more shots and make more trips to the pediatrician than on the conventional schedule. With the timing recommended by the CDC, babies will have five doctor visits in the first fifteen months, and the vaccinations they receive will cover up to fourteen diseases. On one of the most popular delayed schedules, on the other hand, babies will have nine visits in the same amount of time but be immunized against only eight diseases—and still not be covered by that time for measles, rubella, chicken pox, hepatitis A, and hepatitis B. To be clear, an alternative schedule could eventually cover everything; it just takes longer and requires additional trips to the doctor's office, which could create negative associations in the child's mind with visiting the pediatrician.

But the bigger argument against the varying delayed schedules advocated by some is that there's no scientific evidence to support them. At this point there's no proof that an alternative schedule offers positive effects, and one study actually shows that delaying the MMR vaccine beyond fifteen months may increase a baby's seizure risk. The conventional schedule, alternatively, has been carefully calibrated and well researched and is, again, supported by dozens of health organizations and authorities.

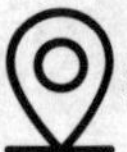

The Bottom Line

WHEN IT COMES to the available scientific research, the evidence is clear. Unless your baby has a medical condition that makes immunization a health risk and you've discussed the pros and cons with your pediatrician, the best course of action is to vaccinate following your physician's guidelines. It's not that immunization is without some risk. It's just that any dangers are so drastically outweighed by the abundant benefits that the decision becomes clear.

The same goes for the CDC-recommended immunization schedule. Delaying vaccinations or using an alternative schedule is better than not immunizing your child at all. But in almost all cases, vaccinations are safe and, when given according to the conventional schedule, will provide babies with the protection they need over their lifetimes to safely navigate their ever-expanding world.

If you prefer an alternative or delayed schedule, make sure you're doing so in coordination with your pediatrician. Or if, despite medical recommendations, your values and beliefs lead you to choose not to vaccinate, inform yourself how best to build your baby's immune system and how to protect your child and the others you'll come into contact with. If you want to read more, both the WHO and the CDC have prepared guides on the risks and responsibilities for families who don't immunize their children.

On a Personal Note

MY HUSBAND AND I didn't have all of this information when our kids were born, so we did the best we could with what we knew. We followed a traditional vaccination schedule with our oldest, but for our two youngest we chose an alternative schedule. They are fully vaccinated, but we stretched out the timetable so they didn't get as many shots at one time. It did mean more visits to the doctor, but at the time we felt better about slowing things down and being a bit more cautious. I don't regret the decision now, and it was one I felt more comfortable with then. Knowing the current state of the research, I would feel fully comfortable going with the traditional vaccine schedule recommended by their pediatrician.

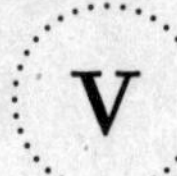

Vaping and Breastfeeding

You know about the dangers of conventional cigarettes, but what about vaping? Is it OK for a nursing mother to vape? Is secondhand smoke an issue?

Competing Opinions

Perspective #1: When you vape, you inhale nicotine, which passes into your breast milk. And even though vaping is different from traditional smoking, it can still affect your baby in negative and serious ways.

Perspective #2: People don't really know enough about vaping yet to say whether it harms a baby or not. But at least it's better than conventional smoking around your infant. And the vapors are much less harmful than those of cigarette smoke.

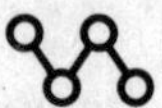

What the Science Says

VAPING IS SUCH a recent phenomenon that the science exploring its effects is still only emerging. At the time of this writing, news has broken regarding new dangers associated with vaping in general. Mysterious and serious lung diseases are being linked to the use of e-cigarettes. Much more research will emerge over the coming months and years.

And still, despite the recency of vaping's popularity, health organizations have had time to weigh in with official, preliminary positions. The AAP has said that vaping during breastfeeding is "risky," and the CDC doesn't even distinguish between conventional and electronic cigarettes and their effect on breastfeeding, warning that "using tobacco or e-cigarettes while breastfeeding can allow harmful chemicals to pass from the mother to the infant through breast milk or secondhand smoke exposure."

We do know that electronic cigarettes, or e-cigarettes, usually contain nicotine, which passes into breast milk and can negatively affect lactation as well as the sleep patterns of infants. This is especially problematic in that e-cigarettes are largely unregulated, meaning that the nicotine dose can vary widely or, as stated in a report from the U.S. Surgeon General, fail to even match what the label says. A recent study out of Australia found that six out of ten e-liquids used in e-cigarettes marketed as nicotine-free actually did contain nicotine. In other words, because of the lack of meaningful regulation, you can't even know exactly what you're ingesting when you vape. Plus, e-cigarettes contain other toxins as well, and research has hardly begun exploring the effects—both short- and long-term—these chemicals might have on developing children.

The other main danger with e-cigarettes when it comes to infants is secondhand vapor. Two different studies have found passive exposure to nicotine via e-cigarettes to be similar to being exposed to conventional cigarettes. Another study found that particulates from secondhand e-cigarette vapor can last in high concentration in a room for more than thirty minutes.

Also potentially risky is what's called "thirdhand smoke," which refers to the residual nicotine and other chemicals that end up on furniture and other surfaces in rooms where smoking has taken place. People can be exposed to these contaminated surfaces by touching them or breathing in the "off-gassing" of what's left behind. Studies haven't linked a similar thirdhand effect to e-cigarettes yet, but as the Surgeon General's report said, it "would be of particular concern for children living in homes of e-cigarette users," since kids crawl on the floor, play in areas where dust can be stirred up, and often put found objects in their mouths.

One final relevant question has to do with whether a mother who smokes, either conventionally or with electronic cigarettes, should stop nursing. As I covered in the "Smoking and Breastfeeding" entry, experts and health organizations—for instance, the AAP and the CDC—agree that the answer is no. You should definitely keep breastfeeding. Obviously, it would be better if you didn't smoke at all, or at least cut down on your smoking. But if you can't quit, you should still breastfeed. Not only will your baby get all of the benefits nursing affords in any situation—the phrase that comes up again and again in the research is that breast milk is the "ideal food" for a baby—there's even evidence that it will also help counteract some of the effects of your smoking or vaping. As the CDC put it in a 2018 statement, "Mothers who use tobacco or e-cigarettes should be encouraged to quit; regardless, breastfeeding provides numerous health benefits and breast milk remains the recommended food for an infant."

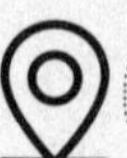

The Bottom Line

MUCH MORE RESEARCH is needed before we can even begin to understand the overall effects of vaping. But the information we do have at the moment paints a clear picture that answers the two key questions: it's not safe to vape while simultaneously nursing, and secondhand vapor from e-cigarettes is absolutely dangerous. If you have the ability to avoid e-cigarettes completely (and conventional cigarettes as well, obviously), do it. If you've never started, don't start now. If you currently vape but can quit for several months, then quit. And before you start up again, check the science to see what new information may have recently emerged.

If you're a vaper or smoker who's unable to kick the habit, you should still nurse your baby and give her the many advantages that come with it, possibly even offsetting some of the negative consequences she'll face as a result of your vaping or smoking. Just be as smart as you can around the issue. Don't smoke or vape while you're nursing, and don't do it near your baby. Smoke or vape immediately after you've nursed, so the nicotine has longer to work itself out of your system before the next feeding, and do it outside to avoid thirdhand smoke in your home or car. If you have the option, consider changing your clothes before holding your baby, so she doesn't experience the thirdhand effects. And most of all, keep trying to quit. It's not easy, and it often takes people several tries before they succeed. But stay at it.

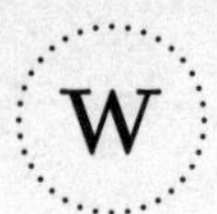

Walkers

Baby walkers have gotten a bad rap over the last several years. Are they really that dangerous?

Competing Opinions

Perspective #1: The AAP has called for an outright ban on walkers for a reason. The dangers include, for example, having babies roll down a flight of stairs, trip and fall over, or maneuver themselves into a position where they could reach something they might not otherwise be able to access—such as a hot stove, a knife, or a household poison. Walkers can even cause developmental delays, keeping kids from crawling and learning how to walk as quickly.

Perspective #2: Walkers are like training wheels on a bike: they offer a great intermediate step toward an important goal. They used to be more dangerous, but the industry has put in place many safety measures—like mandating a width that keeps babies from going through doorways and special sensors that keep them from falling down stairs—and research shows that the number of walker-related injuries is now decreasing. With adequate supervision, there's no reason not to give kids this fun experience that puts them on their way to walking.

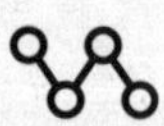

What the Science Says

THE RISKS ASSOCIATED with baby walkers are so significant that the AAP has not only called for a ban on them but also advised parents to throw out any walkers they already have. Numerous studies support the claim that the once-popular parenting item is extremely dangerous on a broad scale. A recent investigation found that almost a quarter of a million U.S.

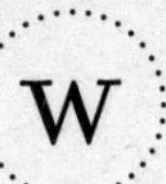

children under fifteen months were treated for walker-related injuries between 1990 and 2014. Most of these were to the head or neck, with the vast majority of injuries incurred from falling down the stairs in the walker. More than a third of the children admitted to the hospital had a skull fracture.

The somewhat-good news is that in 2010, federal mandatory safety standards were put in place for the manufacture of walkers, and over the next few years the average number of injuries decreased by almost 23 percent. What keeps this news only somewhat good, obviously, is that the decrease hasn't been larger. As the authors of the 2018 study put it, "Infant walkers remain an important and preventable source of injury among young children."

The other claim opponents make concerns developmental delays when children don't get the necessary time to crawl and develop the various motor skills that would typically emerge if they weren't spending lots of time speeding around in a walker. While certain methodological concerns have been expressed about the research supporting this claim, it is true that studies have found that walking-related motor development can be slowed by the use of infant walkers.

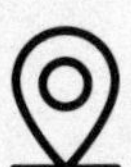

The Bottom Line

IT'S NOT A good idea to put your baby in a walker. Even if you're highly conscientious and vigilant, all parents can get distracted or look away at the wrong time. Instead, consider getting one of the stationary activity centers that let your child spin, bounce, ring bells, and be active in fun ways that won't allow him to hurt himself. Even then, don't become too reliant on the bouncing, rotating devices. Give your child plenty of time on all fours, exercising body and brain as he figures out how to scoot around, crawl, pull himself up, and eventually walk.

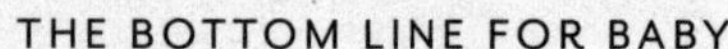

On a Personal Note

WE DIDN'T USE walkers when our children were babies, but we did have a stationary activity center that allowed them to pull levers, manipulate objects, bounce, and rock back and forth. For one of our kids, his favorite activity was spinning. ("Rotating" isn't a strong enough word to describe the high-speed, almost violent circular motion he regularly practiced in his "saucer.") He loved spinning so fast and so much that I became worried and actually called the company who manufactured it! They assured me it was fine. (What else were they going to say?) It makes me wonder whether any baby-product companies keep logs of the oddest crazy-parent calls and questions. I just might be on that list.

The Bottom Line of *The Bottom Line*

If you've stumbled across this book while sitting on the floor in some bookstore, or while searching bleary-eyed through blogs and articles for an answer to whether it's OK to use bug spray on your baby for your summer outing tomorrow: take heart. Yes, you've been given the monumental task of raising this little one who's been entrusted to your care. It's wonderful. But it's also confusing. And scary. And overwhelming. I know. There are *so* many decisions to make about *so* many things. Some are controversial, some seem trivial, and especially when it's your first time making choices for your baby, almost all of the decisions can seem vitally important. You worry that if you choose poorly, it will impact how well your child turns out.

Because we care so much, the stakes feel so high. But we can easily get swept into parenting by fear, getting carried away, living in anxiety, and becoming distracted from what really matters. If you're like me, you sometimes give in to catastrophic thinking. You might begin by worrying that if you don't handle tummy time perfectly, your child will fall behind developmentally. Then you start making mental leaps about problems in school and self-esteem issues, and before long your beautiful infant lying beside you full of promise has turned into a future dropout living in a van down by the river.

So here's the bottom line of *The Bottom Line:* You really can parent well, doing it in a way that helps your infant do more than just survive. You're not alone in being fearful about this little life you're in charge of; virtually all parents feel the same. But you can leave that fear aside, gather information, then listen to what love tells you to do. Yes, you'll make mistakes along the way. Plenty of them. We all do. And no, you won't be able to follow every recommendation in this book in a way that's perfectly consistent with what science and the experts say. But by using the evidence provided here, you can at least make more informed, intentional, and confident decisions about how you parent. Few priorities are more important—for our children, for our families, for our society, for our world—than that we be intentional about the way we raise our kids. The better we understand the bottom line regarding the decisions we're making when our children are young, the better we can do just that.

And remember: it all comes back to relationship. Decades of research have shown that what your baby needs most in order to turn out well is, in fact, *you*. One of the single-most-important predictors for children's outcomes in terms of emotional, social, academic, and career success is that they have secure attachment with at least one caregiver. How do you develop that security in your child? By prioritizing seeing your baby's needs, both physical and emotional, then responding quickly and sensitively so they can learn to trust and to thrive. In the end, your relationship with your child is what matters most.

Acknowledgments

A book like this doesn't come together through the efforts of just one person. I've had lots of help, and I'm grateful to the many people who lent their time, energy, and expertise to the process. Laurel Venne and Claire Penn spent hours helping me research and summarize the findings on the various topics presented here. Alex Van Fleet, Hanna Bogen Novak, and Jamie Chaves provided valuable feedback as pediatric clinicians who are also parents of young children. Scott Bryson, my husband, gave countless hours by being a patient and brilliant editor, helping me dream, think, plan, organize, and edit every word of this book.

Among the many child-development experts, pediatricians, friends, colleagues, and other professionals whose guidance I leaned on, helping me hone and clarify the ideas and make the information as clear and accurate as possible, are Elizabeth Olson, Chris Wolfe, Deborah Buckwalter, Jennifer Shim Lovers, Robyn Park, Chelsey Overstreet, Ross and Carolina Lipstein, Laura Jana, Rob and Catherine Burchell, Joanne Asuncion, Melissa Sprinstead Cahill, Ophelia Chen, Olivia Martinez-Hauge, Roger Thompson, Michael Thompson, and Annemarie Fanselau. In addition, I've relied on researchers and colleagues around the world who have graciously offered their time and expertise to weigh in on the science presented here. Among them are Galen Buckwalter, Scott E. LePor, Maryanne Tigchelaar Perrin, Jenny Radesky, Brian J. Morris, Louisa Gibson, Wendy Goldberg, Maija Bruun Haastrup, Liz Gershoff, Jill Castle, and Fern R. Hauck.

I also want to thank my editor at Random House, Marnie Cochran. Sitting in a booth over lunch, she encouraged me to write a book that I wanted to write, but was afraid to, one that was very different from my typical writing. Marnie has helped me shape the ideas for this book, and her brilliant guidance and encouragement throughout the process mean the world to me. I love getting to work with her and am grateful to have her in my life. And as always, I appreciate my good friend and agent, Doug Abrams. I count on his wisdom and counsel, and I'm especially appreciative of his staff at Idea Architects, in particular Katherine Vaz, whose editorial feedback improved this manuscript in significant ways. I appreciate all that Sarah Breivogel and Colleen Nuccio did to help get this book out to the world.

Finally, I thank Scott and our three boys, for all the ways they support me and keep me grounded while the five of us "do family" and prioritize our relationships with one another, making sure that love remains, always, our bottom line.

Bibliography

What follows is a sample of the sources I used in gathering the information for this book. You can find the complete bibliography at tinabryson.com/bottom-line-bibliography.

Alcohol and Breastfeeding

AAP. (2012). Breastfeeding and the use of human milk. *Pediatrics,* 129 (3), e827–e841.

CDC. (Last reviewed 2018). Alcohol. Centers for Disease Control and Prevention, https://www.cdc.gov/breastfeeding/breastfeeding-special-circumstances/vaccinations-medications-drugs/alcohol.html. Accessed 2019.

Gibson, L., and Porter, M. (2018). Drinking or smoking while breastfeeding and later cognition in children. *Pediatrics,* 142 (2), e20174266.

Haastrup, M. B., et al. (2014). Alcohol and breastfeeding. *Basic and Clinical Pharmacology and Toxicology,* 114 (2), 168–73. This article reviews all evidence available up until the time of its writing, and I highly recommend it.

Mennella, J. A., et al. (2005). Acute alcohol consumption disrupts the hormonal milieu of lactating women. *Journal of Clinical Endocrinology and Metabolism,* 90, 1979–85.

Tay, R. Y., et al. (2017). Alcohol consumption by breastfeeding mothers: Frequency, correlates and infant outcomes. *Drug and Alcohol Review,* 36, 667–76.

Antibiotics

AAP. (Last updated November 15, 2019). Antibiotic prescriptions for children: 10 common questions answered. American Academy of Pediatrics, https://www.healthychildren.org/English/safety-prevention/at-home/medication-safety/Pages/Antibiotic-Prescriptions-for-Children.aspx. Accessed August 2019.

Fleming-Dutra, K. E., et al. (2016). Prevalence of inappropriate antibiotic prescriptions among US ambulatory care visits, 2010–2011. *JAMA,* 315 (17), 1864–73.

Korpela, K., et al. (2016). Intestinal microbiome is related to lifetime antibiotic use in Finnish pre-school children. *Nature Communications,* 7, art. no. 10410.

Nobel, Y., et al. (2015). Metabolic and metagenomic outcomes from early-life pulsed antibiotic treatment. *Nature Communications,* 6, 7486.

Stark, C. M., et al. (2019). Antibiotic and acid-suppression medications during early childhood are associated with obesity. *Gut,* 68 (1), 62–69.

Venekamp, R. P. (2013). Antibiotics for acute otitis media in children. *Cochrane Database of Systemic Reviews,* 1, CD000219.

WHO. (2014). Antimicrobial resistance: Global report on surveillance. World Health Organization, https://apps.who.int/iris/bitstream/handle/10665/112647/WHO_HSE_PED_AIP_2014.2_eng.pdf. Accessed August 2019.

Baby-Led Weaning When Introducing Solids

Brown, A., et al. (2017). Baby-led weaning: The evidence to date. *Current Nutrition Reports,* 6 (2), 148–56. For a thorough examination of current studies on this subject, begin with this paper.

D'Auria, E., et al. (2018). Baby-led weaning: What a systematic review of the literature adds on. *Italian Journal of Pediatrics,* 44 (1), 49.

Dogan, E., et al. (2018). Baby-led complementary feeding: Randomized controlled study. *Pediatrics International,* 60 (12), 1073–80.

Fangupo, L. J., et al. (2016). A baby-led approach to eating solids and risk of choking. *Pediatrics,* 138 (4).

Morison, B. J., et al. (2016). How different are baby-led weaning and conventional complementary feeding? A cross-sectional study of infants aged 6–8 months. *BMJ Open,* 2016 (6), e010665.

Taylor, R. W., et al. (2017). Effect of a baby-led approach to complementary feeding on infant growth and overweight: A randomized clinical trial. *JAMA Pediatrics,* 171 (9), 838–46.

Baby Powder

AAP. (2019). Make baby's room safe: Parent checklist. American Academy of Pediatrics, https://www.healthychildren.org/English/safety-prevention/at-home/Pages/Make-Babys-Room-Safe.aspx. Accessed August 2019.

American Cancer Society. (2018). Talcum powder and cancer, https://www.cancer.org/cancer/cancer-causes/talcum-powder-and-cancer.html. Accessed August 2019.

Murkoff, H., et al. (2019). Should you use talcum powder on your baby? What to expect, https://www.whattoexpect.com/first-year/talcum-powder-for-babies. Accessed August 2019.

Babywearing

Brauer, J., et al. (2016). Frequency of maternal touch predicts resting activity and connectivity of the developing social brain. *Cerebral Cortex,* 26 (8), 3544–52.

Charpak, N., et al. (2017). Twenty-year follow-up of kangaroo mother care versus traditional care. *Pediatrics,* 139 (1).

Conde-Agudelo, A., and Díaz-Rossello, J. L. (2016). Kangaroo mother care to reduce morbidity and mortality in low birthweight infants. *Cochrane Database of Systemic Reviews,* 8 (8).

Esposito, G., et al. (2013). Infant calming responses during maternal carrying in humans and mice. *Current Biology,* 23 (9), 739–45.

USCPSC. (2018). New federal standard to improve safety of infant slings takes effect. United States Consumer Product Safety Commission, https://www.cpsc.gov/content/new-federal-standard-to-improve-safety-of-infant-slings-takes-effect. Accessed August 2019.

Bathing

Jana, L. A., et al. (2015). Baby bath basics. In *Heading Home with Your Newborn: From Birth to Reality*. Elk Grove Village: American Academy of Pediatrics.

Mayo Clinic Staff. (2016). Baby bath basics: A parent's guide. Mayo Clinic, https://www.mayoclinic.org/healthy-lifestyle/infant-and-toddler-health/in-depth/healthy-baby/art-20044438. Accessed August 2019.

Navsaria, D. (2019). Bathing your baby. American Academy of Pediatrics, https://www.healthychildren.org/English/ages-stages/baby/bathing-skin-care/Pages/Bathing-Your-Newborn.aspx. Accessed August 2019.

Ness, M. J., et al. (2013). Neonatal skin care: A concise review. *International Journal of Dermatology,* 52, 14.

Bilingualism

Bialystok, E. (2007). Acquisition of literacy in bilingual children: A framework for research. *Language Learning,* 57 (1), 159–99.

——. (2011). Reshaping the mind: The benefits of bilingualism. *Canadian Journal of Experimental Psychology,* 65 (4), 229–35.

Bialystok, E., et al. (2012). Bilingualism: Consequences for mind and brain. *Trends in Cognitive Science,* 16, 240–50.

Byers-Heinlein, K., et al. (2017). Bilingual infants control their languages as they listen. *Proceedings of the National Academy of Sciences,* 114 (34), 9032–37.

Comishen, K. J., et al. (2019). The impact of bilingual environments on selective attention in infancy. *Developmental Science,* 22 (4), http://babylab.cvr.yorku.ca/files/2019/02/Bilingual-paper.pdf. Accessed August 2019.

Bottles and BPA

AAP. (2012). Baby bottles and bisphenol A (BPA). American Academy of Pediatrics, https://www.healthychildren.org/English/ages-stages/baby/feeding-nutrition/pages/baby-bottles-and-Bisphenol-A-BPA.aspx. Accessed August 2019.

——. (2018). American Academy of Pediatrics says some common food additives may pose health risks to children. American Academy of Pediatrics, https://www.aap.org/en-us/about-the-aap/aap-press-room/Pages/AAP-Says

-Some-Common-Food-Additives-May-Pose-Health-Risks-to-Children.aspx. Accessed August 2019.

CDC. (2017). Bisphenol A (BPA) factsheet. Centers for Disease Control and Prevention, https://www.cdc.gov/biomonitoring/BisphenolA_FactSheet.html. Accessed August 2019.

ECHA. (2017). MSC unanimously agrees that bisphenol A is an endocrine disruptor. European Chemicals Agency, https://echa.europa.eu/-/msc-unanimously-agrees-that-bisphenol-a-is-an-endocrine-disruptor. Accessed August 2019.

EFSA. (2015). No consumer health risk from bisphenol A exposure. European Food Safety Authority, http://www.efsa.europa.eu/en/press/news/150121. Accessed August 2019.

EPA. (Last updated 2017). Risk management for bisphenol A (BPA). U.S. Environmental Protection Agency, https://www.epa.gov/assessing-and-managing-chemicals-under-tsca/risk-management-bisphenol-bpa. Accessed August 2019.

FDA. (2018). Questions and answers on bisphenol A (BPA) use in food contact applications. U.S. Food and Drug Administration, http://www.fda.gov/Food/IngredientsPackagingLabeling/FoodAdditivesIngredients/ucm355155.htm. Accessed August 2019.

Gore, A. C., et al. (2015). Executive Summary to EDC-2: The Endocrine Society's second scientific statement on endocrine-disrupting chemicals. *Endocrine Reviews,* 36 (6), 593–602.

NIH. (2019). Bisphenol A (BPA). National Institutes of Health, https://www.niehs.nih.gov/health/topics/agents/sya-bpa/index.cfm. Accessed August 2019.

Trasande, L., et al. (2018). Food additives and child health. *Pediatrics,* 142 (2), e20181408.

Breastfeeding vs. Formula-Feeding

AAP. Breastfeeding and the use of human milk. American Academy of Pediatrics, http://aappolicy.aappublications.org. Accessed August 2019.

Bartick, M. C., and Reinhold, A. (2010). The burden of suboptimal breastfeeding in the United States: A pediatric cost analysis. *Pediatrics,* 125, e1048–e1056.

——. (2016). Suboptimal breastfeeding in the United States: Maternal and pediatric health outcomes and costs. *Maternal and Child Nutrition,* 13, e12366.

Flaherman, V. J., et al. (2018). The effect of early limited formula on breastfeeding, readmission, and intestinal microbiota: A randomized clinical trial. *Journal of Pediatrics,* 196, 84–90.

Perrin, M. T., et al. (2017). A longitudinal study of human milk composition in the second year postpartum: Implications for human milk banking. *Maternal and Childhood Nutrition,* 13 (1).

UNICEF. (2018). Infant and young child feeding (IYCF) data. UNICEF, https://data.unicef.org/resources/dataset/infant-young-child-feeding. Accessed August 2019.

WHO. (2019). Infant and young child feeding. World Health Organization, https://www.who.int/en/news-room/fact-sheets/detail/infant-and-young-child-feeding. Accessed August 2019.

Bug Spray

AAP. (Last updated July 2018). Choosing an insect repellent for your child. American Academy of Pediatrics, https://www.healthychildren.org/English/safety-prevention/at-play/Pages/Insect-Repellents.aspx. Accessed August 2019.

CDC. (2019). Environmental hazards and other noninfectious health risks. Centers for Disease Control and Prevention, https://wwwnc.cdc.gov/travel/yellowbook/2020/noninfectious-health-risks/injury-and-trauma. Accessed August 2019.

EPA. (Last updated June 2017). DEET. U.S. Environmental Protection Agency, https://www.epa.gov/insect-repellents/deet. Accessed August 2019.

HHS. (2017). Toxicological profile for DEET (N,N-diethyl-meta-toluamide). U.S. Department of Health and Human Services, https://www.atsdr.cdc.gov/toxprofiles/tp185.pdf. Accessed August 2019.

Interlandi, J. (2019). How safe is DEET? Consumer Reports, https://www.consumerreports.org/insect-repellent/how-safe-is-deet-insect-repellent-safety/. Accessed August 2019. This article presents an excellent summary of what we know about DEET and is a good place to start to get a sense of the latest information.

Car Seats

Hoffman, B. D., et al. (2016). Unsafe from the start: Serious misuse of car safety seats at newborn discharge. *Journal of Pediatrics,* 171, 48–54.

Mayo Clinic Staff. (2019). Car seat safety: Avoid 9 common mistakes, https://www.mayoclinic.org/healthy-lifestyle/infant-and-toddler-health/in-depth/car-seat-safety/art-20043939. Accessed August 2019.

NHTSA. (2017). Find the right seat. National Highway Traffic Safety Association, https://www.nhtsa.gov/campaign/right-seat. Accessed August 2019.

Safe Kids Worldwide. (2019). Ultimate car seat guide, https://www.safekids.org/ultimate-car-seat-guide. Accessed August 2019.

Circumcision

AAP. (2012). Male circumcision. *Pediatrics,* 130 (3), e756–85, https://www.ncbi.nlm.nih.gov/pubmed/22926175. Accessed August 2019.

Bossio, J., et al. A review of the current state of the male circumcision literature. *Journal of Sexual Medicine,* 11 (12), 2847–64.

Boyle, G. (2015). Does male circumcision adversely affect sexual sensation, function, or satisfaction? Critical comment on Morris and Krieger. *Advances in Sexual Medicine,* 5, 7–12.

CDC. (2018). Male circumcision. Centers for Disease Control and Prevention, https://www.cdc.gov/hiv/risk/male-circumcision.html. Accessed August 2019.

CPS. (2018). Newborn male circumcision. Canadian Paediatric Society, https://www.cps.ca/en/documents/position/circumcision. Accessed August 2019.

Dave, S., et al. (2018). Canadian Urological Association guideline on the care of the normal foreskin and neonatal circumcision in Canadian infants (full version). *Canadian Urological Association Journal = Journal de l'Association des urologues du Canada,* 12 (2), E76–E99.

Dekker, R., and Bertone, A. (2019). Evidence and ethics on: Circumcision. Evidence-based birth, https://evidencebasedbirth.com/evidence-and-ethics-on-circumcision. Accessed October 2019. See this summary for a helpful and broad-ranging overview of the evidence and arguments on this topic.

Earp, B. D. (2016). Infant circumcision and adult penile sensitivity: Implications for sexual experience. *Trends in Urology and Men's Health,* 7, 17–21.

Earp, B. D., and Shaw, D. (2017). Cultural bias in American medicine: The case of infant male circumcision. *Journal of Pediatric Ethics,* 1, 8–26.

Ellison, J. S., et al. (2018). Neonatal circumcision and urinary tract infections in infants with hydronephrosis. *Pediatrics,* 142 (1), 1–7.

Frisch, M., and Earp, B. D. (2018). Circumcision of male infants and children as a public health measure in developed countries: A critical assessment of recent evidence. *Global Public Health,* 13 (5), 626–41.

Morris, B. J., et al. (2016). Critical evaluation of unscientific arguments disparaging affirmative infant male circumcision policy. *World Journal of Clinical Pediatrics,* 5 (3), 251–61.

———. (2017). Early infant male circumcision: Systematic review, risk-benefit analysis, and progress in policy. *World Journal of Clinical Pediatrics,* 6 (1), 89–102.

Tobian, A.A.R., et al. (2014). Male circumcision: A globally relevant but under-utilized method for the prevention of HIV and other sexually transmitted infections. *Annual Review of Medicine,* 65, 293–306.

WHO. (2010). Neonatal and child male circumcision: A global review. World Health Organization, https://www.who.int/hiv/pub/malecircumcision/neonatal_child_MC_UNAIDS.pdf. Accessed August 2019.

Co-sleeping

Ball, H. L., and Russell, C. K. (2014). SIDS and infant sleep ecology. *Evolution, Medicine and Public Health,* 2014 (1), 146.

Ball, H. L., and Volpe, L. E. (2013). Sudden infant death syndrome (SIDS) risk reduction and infant sleep location—moving the discussion forward. *Social Science and Medicine,* 79, 84–91.

CDC. (2018). Health effects of secondhand smoke. Centers for Disease Control and Prevention, https://www.cdc.gov/tobacco/data_statistics/fact_sheets/secondhand_smoke/health_effects/index.htm. Accessed August 2019.

———. (2018). Sudden unexpected infant death and sudden infant death syndrome. Centers for Disease Control and Prevention, https://www.cdc.gov/sids/about/index.htm. Accessed August 2019.

Doucleff, M. (2018). Is sleeping with your baby as dangerous as doctors say? NPR, https://www.npr.org/sections/goatsandsoda/2018/05/21/601289695/is-sleeping-with-your-baby-as-dangerous-as-doctors-say. Accessed August 2019.

McKenna J.J., et al. (1993). Infant-parent co-sleeping in an evolutionary perspective: Implications for understanding infant sleep development and the sudden infant death syndrome. *Sleep,* 16(3):263e82.

——. (2007). Mother-infant cosleeping, breastfeeding and sudden infant death syndrome: What biological anthropology has discovered about normal infant sleep and pediatric sleep medicine. *American Journal of Physical Anthropology,* 133e61.

Mohr, C., et al. (2019). Patterns of infant regulatory behaviors in relation to maternal mood and soothing strategies. *Child Psychiatry and Human Development,* 4, 566–79.

Moon, R. Y. (2016). SIDS and other sleep-related infant deaths: Evidence base for 2016 updated recommendations for a safe infant sleeping environment. *Pediatrics,* 138 (5).

Oster, E. (2019). *Cribsheet*. New York: Penguin.

Shimizu, M., and Teti, D. M. (2018). Infant sleeping arrangements, social criticism, and maternal distress in the first year. *Infant and Child Development,* 27 (3), e2080.

U.S. Department of Health and Human Services. (2006). *The health consequences of involuntary exposure to tobacco smoke: A report of the Surgeon General.* Atlanta: U.S. Department of Health and Human Services, Centers for Disease Control and Prevention, National Center for Chronic Disease Prevention and Health Promotion, Office on Smoking and Health.

——. (2014). *The health consequences of smoking—50 years of progress: A report of the Surgeon General*. Atlanta: U.S. Department of Health and Human Services, Centers for Disease Control and Prevention, National Center for Chronic Disease Prevention and Health Promotion, Office on Smoking and Health.

Daycare or Nanny?

Barnett, W. S., et al. (2010). The state of preschool, 2010. National Institute for Early Education Research, http://nieer.org/state-preschool-yearbooks/the-state-of-preschool-2010. Accessed August 2019.

Bassok, D., et al. (2016). Within- and between-sector duality differences in early childhood education and care. *Child Development*, 87 (5), 1627–45.

Gomajee, R., et al. (2018). Early childcare type predicts children's emotional and behavioural trajectories into middle childhood. *Journal of Epidemiology and Community Health*, 72, 1033–43.

Loeb, S., et al. (2007). How much is too much? The influence of preschool centers on children's social and cognitive development. *Economics of Education Review*, 26 (1), 52–66.

Magnuson, K. A., et al. (2007). Does prekindergarten improve school preparation and performance? *Economics of Education Review*, 26 (1), 33–51.

NICHD. (2006). NICHD study of early child care and youth development. National Institute of Child Health and Human Development, https://www.nichd.nih.gov/sites/default/files/publications/pubs/documents/seccyd_06.pdf. Accessed August 2019.

Oster, E. (2019). *Cribsheet*. New York: Penguin.

Deciding to Stay at Home?

Bettinger, E., et al. (2014). Home with Mom: The effects of stay-at-home parents on children's long-run educational outcomes. *Journal of Labor Economics*, 32 (3), 443–67.

Chandola, T., et al. (2019). Are flexible work arrangements associated with lower levels of chronic stress-related biomarkers? A study of 6025 employees in the UK Household Longitudinal Study. *Sociology*, 53 (4), 779–99.

Dunifon, R., et al. (2013). The effect of maternal employment on children's academic performance. NBER Working Paper no. w19364, National Bureau of Economic Research, https://ssrn.com/abstract=2315448. Accessed August 2019.

Ettinger, A. K., et al. (2018). Increasing maternal employment influences child overweight/obesity among ethnically diverse families. *Journal of Family Issues*, 39.

Goldberg, W. A., and Loth, L. R. (Forthcoming). Maternal and paternal employment, effects of. In Benson, J. B. (Ed.), *Encyclopedia of Infant and Early Childhood Development*.

Goldberg, W. A., Prause, J., et al. (2008). Maternal employment and children's achievement in context: A meta-analysis of four decades of research. *Psychological Bulletin*, 134, 77–108.

Harrison, L. J., and Ungerer, J. A. (2002). Maternal employment and infant-mother attachment security at 12 months postpartum. *Developmental Psychology*, 38, 758–73.

Huston, A. C., et al. (2015). Time spent in child care: How and why does it affect social development? *Developmental Psychology*, 51 (5), 621–34.

Jeynes, W. H. (2003). A meta-analysis: The effects of parental involvement on minority children's academic achievement. *Education and Urban Society*, 35 (2), 202–18.

Loeb, S., et al. (2007). How much is too much? The influence of preschool centers on children's social and cognitive development. *Economics of Education Review*, 26, 52–66.

Lucas-Thompson, R. G., et al. (2010). Maternal work early in the lives of children and its distal associations with achievement and behavior problems: A meta-analysis. *Psychological Bulletin*, 136 (6), 915–42. This article represents the place to start if you want a wide-ranging meta-analysis of the research available up until 2010. I have relied on it greatly for my summary.

Magnuson, K. A., et al. (2004). Inequality in preschool education and school readiness. *American Educational Research Journal*, 41, 115–57.

McGinn, K. L., et al. (2019). Learning from Mum: Cross-national evidence linking maternal employment and adult children's outcomes. *Work, Employment and Society*, 33 (3), 374–400. This study is worth mentioning even though it falls outside of the focus here since its primary focus is on how children of working mothers turn out *as adults*. The authors find, for example, that "adult daughters, but not sons, of employed mothers are more likely to be employed and, if employed, are more likely to hold supervisory responsibility, work more hours and earn higher incomes than their peers whose mothers were not employed. In the domestic sphere, sons raised by employed mothers spend more time caring for family members and daughters spend less time on housework."

Mendes, E., et al. (2012). Stay-at-home moms report more depression, sadness, anger. Gallup, https://news.gallup.com/poll/154685/stay-home-moms-report-depression-sadness-anger.aspx. Accessed August 2019.

Oster, E. (2019). *Cribsheet*. New York: Penguin.

Thompson, R. A. (2008). Early attachment and later development: Familiar questions, new answers. In J. Cassidy and P. R. Shaver (Eds.), *Handbook of Attachment: Theory, Research, and Clinical Applications*, 348–65. New York: Guilford Press.

Diapers: Disposable vs. Cloth

Allergy News. (2011). Dyes in diapers can cause skin rash. Health.am, http://www.health.am/allergies/more/dyes_in_diapers_can_cause_skin_rash. Accessed August 2019.

Schwarcz, J. (2017). Diapers: Cloth or disposable. McGill University, Office for Science and Society, https://www.mcgill.ca/oss/article/science-science-everywhere/diapers-cloth-or-disposable. Accessed August 2019.

Diet and Breastfeeding

AAP. (2006). *Breastfeeding Handbook for Physicians*. Elk Grove Village, Ill.: American Academy of Pediatrics.

CDC. (2018). Maternal diet: Diet considerations for breastfeeding mothers. Centers for Disease Control and Prevention, https://www.cdc.gov/breastfeeding/breastfeeding-special-circumstances/diet-and-micronutrients/maternal-diet.html. Accessed August 2019.

Daelemans, S., et al. (2018). Recent advances in understanding and managing infantile colic. *F1000 Research*, 7, 1426.

FDA. (2019). Advice about eating fish: For women who are or might become pregnant, breastfeeding mothers, and young children. U.S. Food and Drug Administration, https://www.fda.gov/food/consumers/advice-about-eating-fish#note1. Accessed August 2019.

Godon, M., et al. (2018). Dietary modifications for infantile colic. *Cochrane Database of Systematic Reviews*, doi:10.1002/14651858.CD011029.pub2. Accessed August 2019.

Haastrup, M. B., et al. (2014). Alcohol and breastfeeding. *Basic and Clinical Pharmacology and Toxicology*, 114 (2), 168–73. This article reviews all evidence available up until the time of its writing.

Harb, T., et al. (2016). Infant colic—what works: A systematic review of interventions for breast-fed infants. *Journal of Pediatric Gastroenterology and Nutrition*, 62 (5), 668–86.

Jeong, G., et al. (2017). Maternal food restrictions during breastfeeding. *Korean Journal of Pediatrics*, 60 (3), 70–76. This article offers an excellent summary of research on this question, along with suggestions based on the science.

Rowicka, G., et al. (2017). Diet and nutritional status of children with cow's milk protein allergy, treated with a milk-free diet. *International Journal of Allergy Medications*, 3, 025.

Discipline

Affrunti, N. W. (2014). Temperament, peer victimization, and nurturing parenting in child anxiety: A moderated mediation model. *Child Psychiatry and Human Development*, 45, 483–92.

Arsenio, W., and Ramos-Marcuse, F. (2014). Children's moral emotions, narratives, and aggression: Relations with maternal discipline and support. *Journal of Genetic Psychology*, 175 (5–6), 528–46.

Choe, D. E., et al. (2013). The interplay of externalizing problems and physical and inductive discipline during childhood. *Developmental Psychology*, 49 (11), 2029–39.

Dewar, G. (2017). Authoritarian parenting: What happens to the kids? Parenting Science, https://www.parentingscience.com/authoritarian-parenting.html. Accessed August 2019. As usual, Gwen Dewar's Parenting Science website is very helpful in addressing this situation.

Guyer, A. E., et al. (2014). Lasting associations between early-childhood temperament and late-adolescent reward-circuitry response to peer feedback. *Development and Psychopathology*, 26, 229–43.

Knafo, A., and Plomin, R. (2008). Prosocial behavior from early to middle childhood: Genetic and environmental influences on stability and change. *Developmental Psychology*, 42 (5), 771–86.

Luyckx, K., et al. (2011). Parenting and trajectories of children's maladaptive behaviors: A 12-year prospective community study. *Journal of Clinical Child and Adolescent Psychology*, 40 (3), 468–78.

Maccoby, E. E. (1992). The role of parents in the socialization of children: An historical overview. *Developmental Psychology*, 28, 1006–17.

Piotrowski, J. T., et al. (2013). Investigating correlates of self-regulation in early childhood with a representative sample of English-speaking American families. *Journal of Child and Family Studies*, 22 (3), 423–36.

Siegel, D. J., and Bryson, T. P. (2011). *The Whole-Brain Child: 12 Revolutionary Strategies to Nurture Your Child's Developing Mind*. New York: Random House.

——. (2014). *No-Drama Discipline: The Whole-Brain Way to Calm the Chaos and Nurture Your Child's Developing Mind*. New York: Bantam.

——. (2018). *The Yes Brain: How to Cultivate Courage, Curiosity, and Resilience in Your Child*. New York: Bantam.

——. (2020). *The Power of Showing Up: How Parental Presence Shapes Who Our Kids Become and How Their Brains Get Wired*. New York: Bantam.

Xiao, S. X., et al. (2018). Parental emotion regulation and preschoolers' prosocial behavior: The mediating roles of parental warmth and inductive discipline. *Journal of Genetic Psychology*, 9, 1–10.

Dream Feeding

Dewar, G. (2018). Dream feeding: An evidence based guide to helping babies sleep longer. Parenting Science, https://www.parentingscience.com/dream-feeding.html. Accessed August 2019. This website is a good source of parenting information grounded in science, and Gwen Dewar does a good job of discussing the issues to consider on this subject.

Paul, I. M., et al. (2016). Responsive parenting intervention and infant sleep. *Pediatrics*, 138 (1), e20160762.

Ear Piercing

AAP. (Last updated June 2007). Avoiding infection after ear piercing. American Academy of Pediatrics, https://www.healthychildren.org/English/health-issues/conditions/ear-nose-throat/pages/Avoiding-Infection-After-Ear-Piercing.aspx. Accessed August 2019.

Macgregor, D. M. (2001). The risks of ear piercing in children. *Scottish Medical Journal,* 46 (1), 9–10.

Parekh, J., and Kokotos, F. (2019). Ear piercing. *Pediatrics in Review,* 40 (1), 49–50.

Poe, S., and Cronin, A. (2014). Health risks associated with tattoos and body piercing. *Journal of Clinical Outcomes Management,* 21 (7), 315–20.

Elimination Communication

Bender, J. M., et al. (2017). Elimination communication: Diaper-free in America. *Pediatrics,* 140 (1).

Dewar, G. (2010). Infant toilet training: An evidence-based guide. Parenting Science, https://www.parentingscience.com/infant-toilet-training.html. Accessed August 2019.

Duong, T. H., et al. (2010). Development of bladder control in the first year of life in children who are potty trained early. *Journal of Pediatric Urology,* 6 (5), 501–5.

Rugolotto, S., et al. (2008). Toilet training started during the first year of life: A report on elimination signals, stool toileting refusal and completion age. *Minerva Pediatrica,* 60 (1), 27–35.

Extended Breastfeeding

Bartick, M. C., and Reinhold, A. (2010). The burden of suboptimal breastfeeding in the United States: A pediatric cost analysis. *Pediatrics,* 125, e1048–56.

Bartick, M. C., Schwarz, E. B., et al. (2016). Suboptimal breastfeeding in the United States: Maternal and pediatric health outcomes and costs. *Maternal and Child Nutrition,* 13, e12366.

Chaffee, B. W., et al. (2017). A longitudinal study of human milk composition in the second year postpartum: Implications for human milk banking. *Maternal and Childhood Nutrition,* 13 (1).

Peres, K. G., et al. (2017). Impact of prolonged breastfeeding on dental caries: A population-based birth cohort study. *Pediatrics,* 140 (1).

Tham, R., et al. (2015). Breastfeeding and the risk of dental caries: A systematic review and meta-analysis. *Acta Paediatrica,* 104 (467), 62–84.

UNICEF. (2018). Infant and young child feeding (IYCF) data, https://data.unicef.org/resources/dataset/infant-young-child-feeding. Accessed August 2019.

Weaver, J. M., et al. (2018). Breastfeeding duration predicts greater maternal sensitivity over the next decade. *Developmental Psychology,* 54 (2), 220–27.

WHO. (2019). Infant and young child feeding. *World Health Organization,* https://www.who.int/en/news-room/fact-sheets/detail/infant-and-young-child-feeding. Accessed August 2019.

First Bath

DiCioccio, H., et al. (2019). Initiative to improve exclusive breastfeeding by delaying the newborn bath. *Journal of Obstetric, Gynecologic and Neonatal Nursing,* 48 (2), 189–96. This recent article contains a broad review of relevant research related to the issue.

Navsaria, D. (2019). Bathing your baby. American Academy of Pediatrics, https://www.healthychildren.org/English/ages-stages/baby/bathing-skin-care/Pages/Bathing-Your-Newborn.aspx. Accessed August 2019.

WHO. (2017). WHO recommendations on newborn health. World Health Organization, https://apps.who.int/iris/bitstream/handle/10665/259269/WHO-MCA-17.07-eng.pdf?sequence=1. Accessed August 2019.

Food Allergens and Early Exposure

Burgess, J. A., et al. (2019). Age at introduction to complementary solid food and food allergy and sensitization: A systematic review and meta-analysis. *Clinical and Experimental Allergy,* doi: 10.1111/cea.13383. Accessed August 2019.

Caffarelli, C., et al. (2018). Solid food introduction and the development of food allergies. *Nutrients,* 10 (11), 1790.

Chan, E. S., et al. (2018). Early introduction of foods to prevent food allergy. *Allergy, Asthma and Clinical Immunology,* 14 (Suppl. 2), 57.

Elizur, A., and Katz, Y. (2016). Timing of allergen exposure and the development of food allergy: Treating before the horse is out of the barn. *Current Opinion in Allergy and Clinical Immunology,* 16 (2), 157–64.

Fewtrell, M., et al. (2017). Complementary feeding: A position paper by the European Society for Pediatric Gastroenterology, Hepatology, and Nutrition (ESPGHAN) Committee on Nutrition. *Journal of Pediatric Gastroenterology and Nutrition,* 64 (1), 119–32.

Fisher, H. R., et al. (2019). Preventing peanut allergy: Where are we now? *Journal of Allergy and Clinical Immunology: In Practice,* 7, 367–73.

Greer, F. R., et al. (2019). The effects of early nutritional interventions on the development of atopic disease in infants and children: The role of maternal dietary restriction, breastfeeding, hydrolyzed formulas, and timing of introduction of allergenic complementary foods. *Pediatrics,* 143 (4), e20190281.

Tham, E. H., et al. (2018). Early introduction of allergenic foods for the prevention of food allergy from an Asian perspective: An Asia Pacific Association of Pediatric Allergy, Respirology and Immunology (APAPARI) consensus statement. *Pediatric Allergy and Immunology,* 29 (1), 18–27.

Togias, A., et al. (2017). Addendum guidelines for the prevention of peanut allergy in the United States: Report of the National Institute of Allergy and Infectious Diseases–sponsored expert panel. *Journal of Allergy and Clinical Immunology,* 139, 29–44.

West, C. (2017). Introduction of complementary foods to infants. *Annals of Nutrition and Metabolism,* 70 (Suppl. 2), 47–54.

Germs

Hesselmar, B., et al. (2013). Pacifier cleaning practices and risk of allergy development. *Pediatrics,* 131 (6), e1829–37.

Lynch, S. V., et al. (2014). Effects of early-life exposure to allergens and bacteria on recurrent wheeze and atopy in urban children. *Journal of Clinical Immunology,* 134 (3), 593–601.e12.

——. (2016). Thumb-sucking, nail-biting, and atopic sensitization, asthma, and hay fever. *Pediatrics,* 138 (2).

Stein, M. M., et al. (2016). Innate immunity and asthma risk in Amish and Hutterite farm children. *New England Journal of Medicine,* 375 (5), 411–21.

Introducing Solid Foods

AAP. (2008). (Last updated 2018). Starting solid foods. American Academy of Pediatrics, https://www.healthychildren.org/English/ages-stages/baby/feeding-nutrition/Pages/Switching-to-Solid-Foods.aspx. Accessed August 2019.

——. (2019). Infant food and feeding. American Academy of Pediatrics, https://www.aap.org/en-us/advocacy-and-policy/aap-health-initiatives/HALF-Implementation-Guide/Age-Specific-Content/Pages/Infant-Food-and-Feeding.aspx. Accessed August 2019.

Burgess, J. A., et al. (2019). Age at introduction to complementary solid food and food allergy and sensitization: A systematic review and meta-analysis. *Clinical and Experimental Allergy,* 49 (6), 754–69.

CDC. (2018). When, what, and how to introduce solid foods. Centers for Disease Control and Prevention, https://www.cdc.gov/nutrition/infantandtoddlernutrition/foods-and-drinks/when-to-introduce-solid-foods.html. Accessed August 2019.

Chan, E. S., et al. (2018). Early introduction of foods to prevent food allergy. *Allergy, Asthma and Clinical Immunology,* 14 (57).

Dogan, E., et al. (2018). Baby-led complementary feeding: Randomized controlled study. *Pediatrics International,* 60 (12), 1073–80.

Elizur, A., and Katz, Y. (2016). Timing of allergen exposure and the development of food allergy: Treating before the horse is out of the barn. *Current Opinion in Allergy and Clinical Immunology,* 16 (2), 157–64.

Fisher, H. R., et al. (2019). Preventing peanut allergy: Where are we now? *Journal of Allergy and Clinical Immunology: In Practice*, 7, 367–73.

West, C. (2017). Introduction of complementary foods to infants. *Annals of Nutrition and Metabolism*, 70 (Suppl. 2), 47–54.

Marijuana and Breastfeeding

Bertrand, K., et al. (2018). Marijuana use by breastfeeding mothers and cannabinoid concentrations in breast milk. *Pediatrics*, 142 (3).

Jansson, L., et al. (2018). Perinatal marijuana use and the developing child. *Journal of the American Medical Association*, 320 (6), 545–46.

Metz, T., et al. (2018). Marijuana use in pregnancy and while breastfeeding. *Obstetrics and Gynecology*, 132 (5), 1198–210.

Reece-Stremtan, S., et al. (2015). ABM Clinical Protocol #21: Guidelines for breastfeeding and substance use or substance use disorder. *Breastfeeding Medicine*, 10 (3).

Ryan, S., et al. (2018). Marijuana use during pregnancy and breastfeeding: Implications for neonatal and childhood outcomes. *Pediatrics*, 142 (3).

Massage

Brauer, J., et al. (2016). Frequency of maternal touch predicts resting activity and connectivity of the developing social brain. *Cerebral Cortex*, 26 (8), 3544–52.

Charpak, N., et al. (2017). Twenty-year follow-up of kangaroo mother care versus traditional care. *Pediatrics*, 139 (1).

Conde-Agudelo, A., and Díaz-Rossello, J. L. (2016). Kangaroo mother care to reduce morbidity and mortality in low birthweight infants. *Cochrane Database of Systemic Reviews*, 8 (8).

Mayo Clinic Staff. (2019). Infant massage: Understand this soothing therapy, https://www.mayoclinic.org/healthy-lifestyle/infant-and-toddler-health/in-depth/infant-massage/art-20047151. Accessed August 2019.

Pados, B. F., and McGlothen-Bell, K. (2019). Benefits of infant massage for infants and parents in the NICU. *Nursing for Women's Health*, 23 (3), 265–71.

Vicente S., et al. (2017). Infant massage improves attitudes toward childbearing, maternal satisfaction and pleasure in parenting. *Infant Behavioral Development*, 49, 114–19.

Medications and Breastfeeding

AAP. (2019). Breastfeeding and medication. American Academy of Pediatrics, https://www.aap.org/en-us/Pages/Breastfeeding-and-Medication.aspx. Accessed August 2019.

CDC. (2018). Prescription medication use. Centers for Disease Control and Prevention, https://www.cdc.gov/breastfeeding/breastfeeding-special-circumstances/vaccinations-medications-drugs/prescription-medication-use.html. Accessed August 2019.

Davanzo, R., et al. (2011). Antidepressant drugs and breastfeeding: A review of the literature. *Breastfeeding Medicine*, 6 (2), 89–98.

Drugs and Lactation Database (LactMed). Bethesda, MD: National Library of Medicine, 2006–, https://www.ncbi.nlm.nih.gov/books/NBK501922. Accessed August 2019.

Kim, D. R., et al. (2014). Pharmacotherapy of postpartum depression: An update. *Expert Opinion on Pharmacotherapy*, 15 (9), 1223–34.

Sachs, H. (2013). The transfer of drugs and therapeutics into human breast milk: An update on selected topics. *Pediatrics*, 132 (3). Sachs's wide-ranging discussion of this subject is an excellent source for information about the many issues at play here.

Music

Arnon S., et al. (2006). Live music is beneficial to preterm infants in the neonatal intensive care unit environment. *Birth*, 33, 131–36.

Gerry, D., et al. (2012). Active music classes in infancy enhance musical, communicative and social development. *Developmental Science*, 15 (3), 398.

Hartling L., et al. (2009). Music for medical indications in the neonatal period: A systematic review of randomized controlled trials. *Archives of Disease in Childhood: Fetal and Neonatal Edition*, 94, F349–54.

Nelson, Carlota. (2019). Baby music: The soundtrack to your child's development. UNICEF, https://www.unicef.org/parenting/child-development/baby-music-soundtrack-to-development. Accessed August 2019.

Trainor, L. J. (2012). Musical experience, plasticity, and maturation: Issues in measuring developmental change using EEG and MEG. *Annals of the New York Academy of Sciences,* 1252 (1), 25.

Wong, P. C. M., et al. (2007). Musical experience shapes human brainstem encoding of linguistic pitch patterns. *Natural Neuroscience,* 10 (4), 420–22.

Nipple Confusion

Zimmerman, E. (2018). Pacifier and bottle nipples: The targets for poor breastfeeding outcomes. *Jornal de Pediatria,* 94 (6), 571–73.

Zimmerman, E., and Thompson, K. (2015). Clarifying nipple confusion. *Journal of Perinatology,* 35, 895–99. See this review, along with Zimmerman's 2018 article (cited above), for a clear explanation of the science on the subject.

Nursing Baby to Sleep

AAP. (2019). Falling asleep at the breast/bottle. American Academy of Pediatrics radio series *A Minute for Kids,* https://www.aap.org/en-us/about-the-aap/aap-press-room/aap-press-room-media-center/Pages/Falling-Asleep-at-the-Breast-Bottle.aspx. Accessed August 2019.

Blunden, S. L., et al. (2011). Behavioural sleep treatments and night time crying in infants: Challenging the status quo. *Sleep Medicine Reviews,* 15 (5), 327–34.

Cohen, A., et al. (2012). Breastfeeding may improve nocturnal sleep and reduce infantile colic: Potential role of breast milk melatonin. *European Journal of Pediatrics,* 4, 729–32.

Dewar, G. (2018). 13 evidence-based tips for getting your baby to sleep: Finding the right infant sleep aid. Parenting Science, https://www.parentingscience.com/infant-sleep-aid.html. Accessed August 2019.

Meltzer, L. J., and Mindell, J. A. (2006). Sleep and sleep disorders in children and adolescents. *Psychiatric Clinics of North America,* 29, 1059–76.

Nevarez, D. (2013). Normal infant sleep: Night nursing's importance. *Psychology Today,* https://www.psychologytoday.com/us/blog/moral-landscapes/201303/normal-infant-sleep-night-nursings-importance. Accessed August 2019.

Nikolopoulou, M., and St. James-Roberts, I. (2003). Preventing sleeping problems in infants who are at risk of developing them. *Archives of Disease in Childhood,* 88, 108–11.

On-Demand vs. Scheduled Feeding

AAP. (2017). Responsive feeding: Set your baby up for healthy growth and development. American Academy of Pediatrics, https://ihcw.aap.org/Documents/Early%20Feeding/Responsive%20Feeding/AAP-ResponsiveFeeding-2017-08-24-CMYK_R1.pdf. Accessed August 2019.

Crosson, D. D., and Pickler, R. H. (2004). An integrated review of the literature on demand feedings for preterm infants. *Advances in Neonatal Care,* 4, 216–25.

Dewar, G. (2017). The best infant feeding schedule: Why babies are better off feeding on cue. Parenting Science, https://www.parentingscience.com/infant-feeding-schedule.html. Accessed August 2019. For an excellent discussion of the issue, see the always helpful Parenting Science website, where Gwen Dewar more fully explains and analyzes many of the ideas presented here.

Dinkevich, E., et al. (2015). Mothers' feeding behaviors in infancy: Do they predict child weight trajectories? *Obesity,* 23 (12), 2470–76.

Disantis, K. I., et al. (2011). The role of responsive feeding in overweight during infancy and toddlerhood: A systematic review. *International Journal of Obesity,* 35, 480–92.

Rodgers, R. F., et al. (2013). Maternal feeding practices predict weight gain and obesogenic eating behaviors in young children: A prospective study. *International Journal of Behavioral Nutrition and Physical Activity,* 10 (24).

Tylka, T. L., et al. (2015). Maternal intuitive eating as a moderator of the association between concern about child weight and restrictive child feeding. *Appetite,* 95, 158–65.

Organic Foods

Forman, J., et al. (2012). Organic foods: Health and environmental advantages and disadvantages. *Pediatrics*, 130, e1406.

Grandjean, P. (2017). Health benefits of organic food, farming outlined in new report. Harvard T. H. Chan School of Public Health, https://www.hsph.harvard.edu/news/features/health-benefits-organic-food-farming-report. Accessed August 2019.

Mie, A., et al. (2017). Human health implications of organic food and organic agriculture: A comprehensive review. *Environmental Health*, 16 (1), 111.

Rahmann, G. (2011). Biodiversity and organic farming: What do we know? *Agriculture and Forestry Research*, 61 (3), 189–208.

Smith-Spangler, C. (2012). Are organic foods safer or healthier than conventional alternatives? A systematic review. *Annals of Internal Medicine*, 157 (5), 348–66.

USDA. (Last updated August 2019). Organic market overview. U.S. Department of Agriculture, https://www.ers.usda.gov/topics/natural-resources-environment/organic-agriculture/organic-market-overview.aspx. Accessed August 2019.

Pacifiers

AAP. (2005). The changing concept of sudden infant death syndrome: Diagnostic coding shifts, controversies regarding the sleeping environment, and new variables to consider in reducing risk. *Pediatrics*, 116 (5), 1245–55.

Barca, L., et al. (2017). Pacifier overuse and conceptual relations of abstract and emotional concepts. *Frontiers in Psychology*, December, doi: 10.3389/fpsyg.2017.02014.

Eidelman, A. I., and Schanler, R. J. (2012). Breastfeeding and the use of human milk. *Pediatrics*, 129 (3).

Hauck, F., et al. (2005). Do pacifiers reduce the risk of sudden infant death syndrome? *Pediatrics*, 116 (5), e716–23.

Jaafar, S. H., et al. (2011). Pacifier use versus no pacifier use in breastfeeding term infants for increasing duration of breastfeeding. *Cochrane Database Systematic Reviews*, 16 (3), CD007202.

Kramer, M., et al. (2001). Pacifier use, early weaning, and cry/fuss behavior: A randomized controlled trial. *JAMA*, 286 (3), 322–26.

Moon, R. (2016). SIDS and other sleep-related infant deaths: Evidence base for 2016 updated recommendations for a safe infant sleeping environment. *Pediatrics*, 138 (5). For an in-depth look at research regarding pacifier use, this article is an excellent place to start.

Niedenthal, P. M. (2012). Negative relations between pacifier use and emotional competence. *Basic and Applied Social Psychology*, 34 (5), 387–94.

Rychlowska, M., et al. (2014). Pacifiers disrupt adults' responses to infants' emotions. *Basic and Applied Social Psychology*, 36 (4), 299–308.

Sexton, S., et al. (2009). Risks and benefits of pacifiers. *American Family Physician*, 79 (8), 681–85.

Shotts, L., et al. (2008). The impact of prolonged pacifier use on speech articulation: A preliminary investigation. *Contemporary Issues in Communication and Disorders*, 35, 72–75.

"Parentese" and Baby Talk

Cristia, A. (2013). Input to language: The phonetics and perception of infant-directed speech. *Language and Linguistics Compass*, 7 (3), 157–70.

Dunst, C. J., et al. (2012). Preference for infant-directed speech in preverbal young children. *CELL Reviews* (Center for Early Literacy Learning), 5 (1).

Elmlinger, S., et al. (2019). The ecology of prelinguistic vocal learning: Parents simplify the structure of their speech in response to babbling. *Journal of Child Language*, 46 (5), 998–1011.

Fernald, A. (1985). Four-month-old infants prefer to listen to motherese. *Infant Behavioral Development*, 8, 181–95.

Madigan, S., et al. (2019). Parenting behavior and child language: A meta-analysis. *Pediatrics*, 144 (4).

Ramírez-Esparza, N., et al. (2017). Look who's talking now! Parentese speech, social context, and language development across time. *Frontiers in Psychology*, 8. For an exhaustive summary of the research on the subject, see this recent article. Many of the other studies cited here dovetail and overlap.

UNICEF. (2018). Master class with Dr. Marina Kalashnikova. YouTube, https://youtube/378xfXr8OWA. Accessed August 2019.

Pets

AACAP. (2019). Pets and children. American Academy of Child and Adolescent Psychiatry, no. 75, https://www.aacap.org/aacap/families_and_youth/facts_for_families/fff-guide/pets-and-children-075.aspx. Accessed August 2019.

Gadomski, A. M., et al. (2015). Pet dogs and children's health: Opportunities for chronic disease prevention? Preventing Chronic Disease, https://www.cdc.gov/pcd/issues/2015/15_0204.htm. Accessed August 2019.

Hurley, K., and Oakes, L. M. (2018). Infants' daily experience with pets and their scanning of animal faces. *Frontiers in Veterinary Science,* 5, 152.

Kovack-Lesh, K. A., et al. (2014). Four-month-old infants' visual investigation of cats and dogs: Relations with pet experience and attentional strategy. *Developmental Psychology,* 50 (2), 402–13.

Lodge, C. J., et al. (2012). Perinatal cat and dog exposure and the risk of asthma and allergy in the urban environment: A systematic review of longitudinal studies. *Clinical Development Immunology,* 2012, 176484.

Tun, H. M., et al. (2017). Exposure to household furry pets influences the gut microbiota of infants at 3–4 months following various birth scenarios. *Microbiome,* 5 (1), 40.

Postpartum Depression

Brock, R. L., et al. (2019). An integrated relational framework of depressed mood and anhedonia during pregnancy. *Journal of Marriage and Family,* 77.

Drugs and Lactation Database (LactMed). Bethesda, MD: National Library of Medicine, 2006–, https://www.ncbi.nlm.nih.gov/books/NBK501922. Accessed August 2019.

Figueiredo, J. A., et al. (2019). Preterm birth as a risk factor for postpartum depression: A systematic review and meta-analysis. *Journal of Affective Disorders,* 259, 392–403.

Inserro, A. (2018). Challenges of treating postpartum depression. AJMC, https://www.ajmc.com/conferences/psychcongress2018/challenges-of-treating-postpartum-depression. Accessed August 2019.

Kim, D. R., et al. (2014). Pharmacotherapy of postpartum depression: An update. *Expert Opinion on Pharmacotherapy,* 15 (9), 1223–34.

Mayo Clinic. (2018). Postpartum depression, https://www.mayoclinic.org/diseases-conditions/postpartum-depression/symptoms-causes/syc-20376617. Accessed August 2019.

Netsi E., et al. (2018). Association of persistent and severe postnatal depression with child outcomes. *JAMA Psychiatry,* 75 (3), 247–53.

O'Hara, M. W., and McCabe, J. E. (2013). Postpartum depression. *Annual Review of Clinical Psychology,* 9 (1), 379–407.

Surkan, P. J., et al. (2014). Early maternal depressive symptoms and child growth trajectories: A longitudinal analysis of a nationally representative US birth cohort. *BMC Pediatrics,* 14, 185.

Woolhouse H., et al. (2016). Maternal depression from pregnancy to 4 years postpartum and emotional/behavioural difficulties in children: Results from a prospective pregnancy cohort study. *Archives of Women's Mental Health,* 19 (1), 141–51.

Yim, I. S., et al. (2015). Biological and psychosocial predictors of postpartum depression: Systematic review and call for integration. *Annual Review of Clinical Psychology,* 11 (1), 99–137.

Potty-Training an Infant

Blum, N. J., et al. (2003). Relationship between age at initiation of toilet training and duration of training: A prospective study. *Pediatrics,* 111 (4, Pt. 1), 810–14.

Dewar, G. (Last updated 2015). The timing of toilet training: What's the best potty training age? Parenting Science, https://www.parentingscience.com/potty-training-age.html. Accessed August 2019.

Hodges, S., et al. (2014). The association of age of toilet training and dysfunctional voiding. *Research and Reports in Urology,* 127.

——. (2017). The dangerous consequences of potty training too early. For Every Mom, https://foreverymom.com/family-parenting/dangers-potty-training-too-early-dr-steve-hodges. Accessed August 2019.

Kimball, V. (2016). The perils and pitfalls of potty training. *Pediatric Annals,* 45 (6), e199–201.

Oster, E. (2019). *Cribsheet*. New York: Penguin.

Schum, T. R., et al. (2002). Sequential acquisition of toilet-training skills: A descriptive study of gender and age differences in normal children. *Pediatrics,* 109, 48–54.

Probiotics

AAP. (2018). Probiotics in infant formula. American Academy of Pediatrics, https://www.healthychildren.org/English/ages-stages/baby/formula-feeding/Pages/Probiotics-in-Infant-Formula.aspx. Accessed August 2019.

Didari, T., et al. (2014). A systematic review of the safety of probiotics. *Expert Opinion on Drug Safety,* 13 (2), 227–39.

NIH. (2019). Probiotics: What you need to know. National Institutes of Health, https://nccih.nih.gov/health/probiotics/introduction.htm. Accessed August 2019.

Quin, C. (2018). Probiotic supplementation and associated infant gut microbiome and health: A cautionary retrospective clinical comparison. *Scientific Reports,* 8, art. no. 8283. This recent article offers an excellent, wide-ranging overview of where research stands on the question of infants and probiotics.

Thomas, D. W., et al. (2010). Probiotics and prebiotics in pediatrics. *Pediatrics,* 126 (6), 1217–31.

Pumped Milk vs. Direct Breastfeeding

Abedi, P., et al. (2016). Breastfeeding or nipple stimulation for reducing postpartum haemorrhage in the third stage of labour. *Cochrane Database of Systemic Reviews,* CD010845, doi: 10.1002/14651858.CD010845.pub2. Accessed August 2019.

Ballard, O., and Morrow, A. L. (2013). Human milk composition: Nutrients and bioactive factors. *Pediatric Clinics of North America,* 60 (1), 49–74.

Cabrera-Rubio, R., et al. (2012). The human milk microbiome changes over lactation and is shaped by maternal weight and mode of delivery. *American Journal of Clinical Nutrition,* 96 (3), 544–51.

Dilli, D., et al. (2009). Interventions to reduce pain during vaccination in infancy. *Journal of Pediatrics,* 154 (3), 385–90.

Ewaschuk, J. B., et al. (2011). Effect of pasteurization on selected immune components of donated human breast milk. *Journal of Perinatology,* 31 (9), 593–98.

Penn, A. (2014). Effect of digestion and storage of human milk on free fatty acid concentration and cytotoxicity. *Journal of Pediatric Gastroenterology and Nutrition,* 59 (3), 365–73.

Rasmussen, K. M., and Geraghty, S. R. (2011). The quiet revolution: Breastfeeding transformed with the use of breast pumps. *American Journal of Public Health,* 101 (8), 1356–59.

Reading to Baby

All experts, everywhere, agree.

Screen Time

AAP. (2016). Media and young minds. *Pediatrics,* 138 (5).

Anderson, D. R., and Pempek, T. A. (2005). Television and very young children. *American Behavioral Scientist,* 48 (5), 505–22.

Courage, M. L., et al. (2016). Infants, toddlers and learning from screen media. *Encyclopedia on Early Childhood Development,* http://www.child-encyclopedia.com/technology-early-childhood-education/according-experts/infants-toddlers-and-learning-screen-media. Accessed August 2019.

Cox, R., et al. (2012). Television viewing, television content, food intake, physical activity and body mass index: A cross-sectional study of preschool children aged 2–6 years. *Health Promotion Journal of Australia,* 23 (1), 58–62.

DeLoache, J. S. (2010). Do babies learn from baby media? *Psychological Science,* 21 (11), 1570–74.

Duch, H., et al. (2013). Screen time use in children under 3 years old: A systematic review of correlates. *International Journal of Behavioral Nutrition and Physical Activity,* 10, 102. This article provides a broad and helpful summary of much of the research related to this topic.

Hinkley, T., et al. (2014). Early childhood electronic media use as a predictor of poorer well-being: A prospective cohort study. *JAMA Pediatrics*, 168 (5), 485–92.

Lin, Y., et al. (2015). Effects of television exposure on developmental skills among young children. *Infant Behavior and Development*, 38, 20–26.

Linebarger, D. L., and Vaala, S. E. (2010). Screen media and language development in infants and toddlers: An ecological perspective. *Developmental Review*, 30 (2), 176–202.

Madigan, S., et al. (2019). Association between screen time and children's performance on a developmental screening test. *JAMA Pediatrics*, 173 (3), 244–50.

Troseth, G. L., et al. (2018). Let's chat: On-screen social responsiveness is not sufficient to support toddlers' word learning from video. *Frontiers in Psychology*, 9, 2195.

van den Heuvel, M., et al. (2019). Mobile media device use is associated with expressive language delay in 18-month-old children. *Journal of Developmental and Behavioral Pediatrics*, 40 (2), 99–104.

Vijakkhana, N., et al. (2015). Evening media exposure reduces night-time sleep. *Acta Paediatrica*, 104 (3), 306–12.

WHO. (2019). Guidelines on physical activity, sedentary behaviour and sleep for children under 5 years of age. World Health Organization, https://apps.who.int/iris/bitstream/handle/10665/311664/9789241550536-eng.pdf?sequence=1&isAllowed=y. Accessed August 2019.

Security Blankets

AAP. (2016). American Academy of Pediatrics announces new safe sleep recommendations to protect against SIDS, sleep-related infant deaths. American Academy of Pediatrics, https://www.aap.org/en-us/about-the-aap/aap-press-room/pages/american-academy-of-pediatrics-announces-new-safe-sleep-recommendations-to-protect-against-sids.aspx. Accessed August 2019.

AAP Task Force on Sudden Infant Death Syndrome. (2016). SIDS and other sleep-related infant deaths: Updated 2016 recommendations for a safe infant sleeping environment. *Pediatrics*, 138 (5), e20162938.

Sedation While Traveling

Callahan, A. (2012). Using Benadryl for travel with a toddler: A cautionary tale and a little science. Science of Mom, https://scienceofmom.com/2012/06/28/using-benadryl-for-travel-with-a-toddler-a-cautionary-tale-and-a-little-science/#_ENREF_3. Accessed August 2019. This article, from Callahan's website, The Science of Mom, offers an honest and funny story about flying with her own infant, then presents a good overview of available research.

Johnson and Johnson. (2016). Benadryl dosing guide, https://www.benadryl.com/benadryl-dosing-guide. Accessed August 2019.

Nierengarten, M. (2016). Kids on planes. *Contemporary Pediatrics*, 33 (5), 26–28. See this article for a slightly more recent summary of the issue from a pediatrician's point of view.

Sensitive Babies

Calkins, S. D., and Degnan, K. A. (2006). Temperament in early development. In Ammerman, R. (Ed.), *Comprehensive Handbook of Personality and Psychopathology, Vol. 3: Child Psychopathology*. New York: Wiley.

Guyer, A. E., et al. (2015). Temperament and parenting styles in early childhood differentially influence neural response to peer evaluation in adolescence. *Journal of Abnormal Child Psychology,* 43 (5), 863–74.

McLeod, B. D., et al. (2007). Examining the association between parenting and childhood anxiety: A meta-analysis. *Clinical Psychology Review,* 27, 155–72.

Propper, C., and Moore, G. A. (2006). The influence of parenting on infant emotionality: A multi-level psychobiological perspective. *Developmental Review,* 26, 427–60.

Rubin, K. H., and Burgess, K. (2002). Parents of aggressive and withdrawn children. In Bornstein, M., (Ed.), *Handbook of Parenting, Vol. 1,* 383–418. Hillsdale, NJ: Lawrence Erlbaum Associates.

Van Leeuwen, K. G., et al. (2004). Child personality and parental behavior as moderators of problem behavior: Variable- and person-centered approaches. *Developmental Psychology,* 40, 1028–46.

Wood, J. J., et al. (2003). Parenting and childhood anxiety: Theory, empirical findings, and future directions. *Journal of Child Psychology, Psychiatry, and Allied Disciplines,* 44, 134–51.

Sign Language

Fitzpatrick, E., et al. (2014). How HANDy are baby signs? A systematic review of the impact of gestural communication on typically developing, hearing infants under the age of 36 months. *First Language,* 34 (6), 486–509.

Goodwyn, S. W., et al. (2000). Impact of symbolic gesturing on early language development. *Journal of Nonverbal Behavior,* 24, 81–103.

Howard, L., and Doherty-Sneddon, G. (2014). How HANDy are baby signs? A commentary on a systematic review of the impact of gestural communication on typically developing, hearing infants under the age of 36 months. *First Language,* 34 (6), 510–15.

Johnston, J., et al. (2005). Teaching gestural signs to infants to advance child development. *First Language,* 25 (2), 235–51.

Mueller, V., et al. (2014). The effects of baby sign training on child development. *Early Child Development and Care,* 184, 1178–91.

Seal, B. (2010). About baby signing. *ASHA Leader,* doi: 10.1044/leader.FTR5.15132010.np. Accessed August 2019.

Thompson, R. H., et al. (2007). Enhancing early communication through infant sign training. *Journal of Applied Behavior Analysis,* 40 (1), 15–23.

Vallotton, C. D., and Ayoub, C. C. (2010). Symbols build communication and thought: The role of gestures and words in the development of engagement skills and social-emotional concepts during toddlerhood. *Social Development,* 19 (3), 601–26.

Silence vs. Noise in the House

AAP. (2014). Can infant sleep machines be hazardous to babies' ears? American Academy of Pediatrics, https://www.aap.org/en-us/about-the-aap/aap-press

-room/Pages/Can-Infant-Sleep-Machines-Be-Hazardous-to-Babies%27-Ears .aspx. Accessed August 2019.

ASHA. (1997–2019). Loud noise dangers. American Speech-Language-Hearing Association, https://www.asha.org/public/hearing/Loud-Noise-Dangers. Accessed August 2019.

Hugh, S. C., et al. (2014). Infant sleep machines and hazardous sound pressure levels. *Pediatrics,* 133 (4), 677–81.

Mahboubi, H., et al. (2013). Systematic assessment of noise amplitude generated by toys intended for young children. *Otolaryngology—Head and Neck Surgery,* 148 (6), 1043–47.

Sleep Training

Dewar, G. (2016). Gentle infant sleep training. Parenting Science, https://www .parentingscience.com/infant-sleep-training.html. Accessed August 2019.

——. (2017). The Ferber method: What is it, and how does it affect babies? Parenting Science, https://www.parentingscience.com/Ferber-method.html. Accessed August 2019.

Eckerberg, B. (2004). Treatment of sleep problems in families with young children: Effects of treatment on family well-being. *Acta Paediatrica,* 93 (1), 126–34.

Ferber, R. (2006). *Solving Your Child's Sleep Problems: New, Revised, and Expanded Edition.* New York: Fireside.

Gradisar, M., et al. (2016). Behavioral interventions for infant sleep problems: A randomized controlled trial. *Pediatrics,* 137 (6), e20151486.

Hall, W. A., et al. (2015). A randomized controlled trial of an intervention for infants' behavioral sleep problems. *BMC Pediatrics,* 15, 181.

Higley, E., and Dozier, M. (2009). Nighttime maternal responsiveness and infant attachment at one year. *Attachment and Human Development,* 11(4), 347–63.

Hiscock, H., et al. (2007). Improving infant sleep and maternal mental health: A cluster randomized trial. *Archives of Disease in Childhood,* 92 (11), 952–58.

Honaker, S., et al. (2018). Real-world implementation of infant behavioral sleep interventions: Results of a parental survey. *Journal of Pediatrics,* 199, 106–11.e2.

Korownyk, C., and Lindblad, A. J. (2018). Infant sleep training: Rest easy? *Canadian Family Physician,* 64 (1), 41. See this article for a quick and helpful rundown of the research available on the subject.

Lyons, D. M., et al. (2010). Animal models of early life stress: Implications for understanding resilience. *Developmental Psychobiology,* 52 (5), 402–10.

Matthey, S., and Črnčec, R. (2012). Comparison of two strategies to improve infant sleep problems, and associated impacts on maternal experience, mood and infant emotional health: A single case replication design study. *Early Human Development,* 88 (6), 437–42.

Mindell, J. A., et al. (2006). Behavioral treatment of bedtime problems and night wakings in infants and young children. *Sleep,* 29 (10), 1263–76. Erratum: *Sleep,* 29 (11), 1380.

Narvaez, D. (2016). Flawed sleep-training study makes invalid claims. *Psychology Today,* https://www.psychologytoday.com/us/blog/moral-landscapes/201606/flawed-sleep-training-study-makes-invalid-claims-in-the-news. Accessed August 2019.

Philbrook, L.E., et al. (2014). Maternal emotional availability at bedtime and infant cortisol at 1 and 3 months. *Early Human Development,* 90, 595–605.

Price, A.M.H., et al. (2012). Five-year follow-up of harms and benefits of behavioral infant sleep intervention: Randomized trial. *Pediatrics,* 130 (4), 643–51.

Teti, D. M., et al. (2010). Maternal emotional availability at bedtime predicts infant sleep quality. *Journal of Family Psychology,* 24(3), 307–315.

Sleeping in Car Seats, Swings, and Strollers

CDC. (2019). Helping babies sleep safely. Centers for Disease Control and Prevention, https://www.cdc.gov/reproductivehealth/features/baby-safe-sleep/index.html. Accessed August 2019.

Hohman, M. (2016). What you need to know about letting baby sleep in a car seat. What to Expect, https://www.whattoexpect.com/wom/baby/1105/what-you-need-to-know-about-letting-baby-sleep-in-a-car-seat. Accessed August 2019.

Liaw, P., et al. (2019). Infant deaths in sitting devices. *Pediatrics,* 144 (1), e20182576.

Wyckoff, A. S. (2019). Large study sheds light on infant deaths in sitting devices. *AAP News,* May 20, https://www.aappublications.org/news/2019/05/20/sittingdevices052019. Accessed August 2019.

Smoking and Breastfeeding

AAP. (2019). Breastfeeding. American Academy of Pediatrics, https://www.aap.org/en-us/advocacy-and-policy/aap-health-initiatives/Breastfeeding/Pages/Benefits-of-Breastfeeding.aspx. Accessed August 2019.

Banderali, G., et al. (2015). Short and long term health effects of parental tobacco smoking during pregnancy and lactation: A descriptive review. *Journal of Translational Medicine,* 13, 327.

Batstra, L., et al. (2003). Can breast feeding modify the adverse effects of smoking during pregnancy on the child's cognitive development? *Journal of Epidemiology and Community Health,* 57, 403–4.

Bonyata, Kelly. (2018). Breastfeeding and cigarette smoking. Kelly Mom, https://kellymom.com/bf/can-i-breastfeed/lifestyle/smoking. Accessed August 2019.

CDC. (2018). Health effects of secondhand smoke.

——. (2018). Tobacco and e-cigarettes. Centers for Disease Control and Prevention, https://www.cdc.gov/breastfeeding/breastfeeding-special-circumstances/vaccinations-medications-drugs/tobacco-and-e-cigarettes.html. Accessed August 2019.

Gibson, L., and Porter, M. (2018). Drinking and smoking while breastfeeding and later cognition in children. *Pediatrics,* 142 (2), e20174266. This article provides a broad overview of the science surrounding the issues of drinking and smoking while breastfeeding.

Hayes, J. T. (2017). What is thirdhand smoke, and why is it a concern? Mayo Clinic, https://www.mayoclinic.org/healthy-lifestyle/adult-health/expert-answers/third-hand-smoke/faq-20057791. Accessed August 2019.

La Leche League. (2019). Smoking and breastfeeding, https://www.llli.org/breastfeeding-info/smoking-and-breastfeeding/. Accessed August 2019.

SCOTH. (2016). Secondhand smoke: Review of the evidence since 1998. Update of evidence on health effects of secondhand smoke. Scientific Committee on Tobacco and Health, http://www.smokefreeengland.co.uk/files/scoth_secondhandsmoke.pdf. Accessed August 2019.

U.S. Department of Health and Human Services. (2014). *Surgeon General's report: The health consequences of smoking: 50 years of progress*, https://www.cdc.gov/tobacco/data_statistics/sgr/50th-anniversary/index.htm. Accessed August 2019.

Social Media and Your Baby's Online Presence

Brosch, A. (2016). When the child is born into the Internet: Sharenting as a growing trend among parents on Facebook. *New Educational Review*, 43, 225–35. This article is the place to begin to see an excellent summary of the available research.

Fox, A. K., and Hoy, M. G. (2019). Smart devices, smart decisions? Implications of parents' sharenting for children's online privacy: An investigation of mothers. *Journal of Public Policy and Marketing*.

Steinberg, S. (2017). Sharenting: Children's privacy in the age of social media. *Emory Law Journal*, 66, 839.

University of Tennessee at Knoxville. (2019). New moms may be vulnerable to "sharenting." *Science Daily*, July 23, https://www.sciencedaily.com/releases/2019/07/190723121900.htm. Accessed August 2019.

Verswijvel, K., et al. (2019). Sharenting, is it a good or a bad thing? Understanding how adolescents think and feel about sharenting on social network sites. *Children and Youth Services Review*, 104, 319–27.

Spanking

Afifi, T. O., et al. (2017). The relationships between harsh physical punishment and child maltreatment in childhood and intimate partner violence in adulthood. *BMC Public Health*, 17 (1), 493.

——. (2017). Spanking and adult mental health impairment: The case for the designation of spanking as an adverse childhood experience. *Child Abuse and Neglect*, 71, 24–31.

APA. (2019). Resolution on physical discipline of children by parents. American Psychological Association, https://www.apa.org/about/policy/physical-discipline.pdf. Accessed August 2019.

——. (2019). Task force on physical punishment of children. American Psychological Association, https://www.apadivisions.org/division-37/news-events/hitting-children. Accessed August 2019.

Cole, D. (2018). What happens when a country bans spanking? NPR, October 25, https://www.npr.org/sections/goatsandsoda/2018/10/25/660191806/what-happens-when-a-country-bans-spanking. Accessed August 2019.

Felitti, V. J., et al. (1998). Relationship of childhood abuse and household dysfunction to many of the leading causes of death in adults. The Adverse Childhood Experiences (ACE) Study. *American Journal of Preventive Medicine,* 14 (4), 245–58.

Ferguson, C. J. (2013). Spanking, corporal punishment and negative long-term outcomes: A meta-analytic review of longitudinal studies. *Clinical Psychology Review,* 33, 196–208.

Fortson, B. L., et al. (2016). Preventing child abuse and neglect: A technical package for policy, norm, and programmatic activities. Centers for Disease Control and Prevention, https://www.cdc.gov/violenceprevention/pdf/can-prevention-technical-package.pdf. Accessed August 2019.

Gershoff, E. T. (2002). Corporal punishment by parents and associated child behaviors and experiences: A meta-analytic and theoretical review. *Psychological Bulletin,* 128, 539–79.

Gershoff, E. T., and Grogan-Kaylor, A. (2016). Spanking and child outcomes: Old controversies and new meta-analyses. *Journal of Family Psychology,* 30 (4), 453–69.

Gershoff, E. T., Sattler, K. M. P., and Ansari, A. (2018). Strengthening causal estimates for links between spanking and children's externalizing behavior problems. *Psychological Science,* 29 (1), 110–20.

Holden, G. W., et al. (2017). Researchers deserve a better critique: Response to Larzelere, Gunnoe, Roberts, and Ferguson (2017). *Marriage and Family Review,* 53 (5), 465–90.

Larzelere, R. E., and Kuhn, B. R. (2005). Comparing child outcomes of physical punishment and alternative disciplinary tactics: A meta-analysis. *Clinical Child and Family Psychology Review,* 8, 1–37.

——. (Last updated April 2016). Comparing child outcomes of physical punishment and alternative disciplinary tactics: A meta-analysis (Larzelere & Kuhn, 2005): Major conclusions and comparisons with other meta-analyses through 2016, College of Human Sciences, Oklahoma State University, https://humansciences.okstate.edu/hdfs/directory/images/larzelere-kuhn-2005.pdf. Accessed August 2019.

MacKenzie, M. J., et al. (2015). Spanking and children's externalizing behavior across the first decade of life: Evidence for transactional processes. *Journal of Youth and Adolescence,* 44 (3), 658–69.

Sege, R., and Siegel, B. (2018). Effective discipline to raise healthy children. *Pediatrics,* 142.

Siegel, D. J., and Bryson, T. P. (2014). *No-Drama Discipline: The Whole-Brain Way to Calm the Chaos and Nurture Your Child's Developing Mind*. New York: Bantam.

Streit, C., et al. (2017). Negative emotionality and discipline as long-term predictors of behavioral outcomes in African American and European American children. *Developmental Psychology,* 53 (6), 1013–26.

Tomoda, A., et al. (2009). Reduced prefrontal cortical gray matter volume in young adults exposed to harsh corporal punishment. *NeuroImage,* 47 (Suppl. 2), T66–71.

Wang, M., and Liu, L. (2018). Reciprocal relations between harsh discipline and children's externalizing behavior in China: A 5-year longitudinal study. *Child Development,* 89 (1), 174–87.

Spoiling a Baby by Too Much Holding

Benoit, D. (2004). Infant-parent attachment: Definition, types, antecedents, measurement and outcome. *Paediatrics and Child Health,* 9 (8), 541–45.

Charpak, N. (2017). Twenty-year follow-up of kangaroo mother care versus traditional care. *Pediatrics,* https://pediatrics.aappublications.org/content/pediatrics/139/1/e20162063.full.pdf. Accessed August 2019.

Conde-Agudelo, A., and Díaz-Rossello, J. L. (2016). Kangaroo mother care to reduce morbidity and mortality in low birthweight infants. *Cochrane Database Systematic Reviews,* CD 002771, doi: 10.1002/14651858.CD002771.pub4.

Gray, L., et al. (2012). Skin-to-skin contact is analgesic in healthy newborns. *Pediatrics,* 105 (1), e14.

Hong, Y. R., and Park, J. S. (2012). Impact of attachment, temperament and parenting on human development. *Korean Journal of Pediatrics,* 55 (12), 449–54.

Moore, E. R., et al. (2012). Early skin-to-skin contact for mothers and their healthy newborn infants. *Cochrane Database Systematic Reviews,* CD 003519, https://www.cochrane.org/CD003519/PREG_early-skin-skin-contact-mothers-and-their-healthy-newborn-infants. Accessed August 2019.

Sroufe, L. A. (2005). Attachment and development: A prospective, longitudinal study from birth to adulthood. *Attachment and Human Development,* 7, 349–67.

Sullivan, R., et al. (2012). Infant bonding and attachment to the caregiver: Insights from basic and clinical science. *Clinics in Perinatology,* 38 (4), 643–55.

Vittner, D., et al. (2018). Increase in oxytocin from skin-to-skin contact enhances development of parent-infant relationship. *Biological Research for Nursing,* 20 (1), 54–62.

Stranger Anxiety

Guyer, A. E., et al. (2015). Temperament and parenting styles in early childhood differentially influence neural response to peer evaluation in adolescence. *Journal of Abnormal Child Psychology,* 43 (5), 863–74.

Matsuda, Y. T., et al. (2013). Shyness in early infancy: Approach-avoidance conflicts in temperament and hypersensitivity to eyes during initial gazes to faces. *PLOS One,* 8 (6), e65476.

Propper, C., and Moore, G. A. (2006). The influence of parenting on infant emotionality: A multi-level psychobiological perspective. *Developmental Review,* 26, 427–60.

Putnam, S. P., and Stifter, C. A. (2002). Development of approach and inhibition in the first year: Parallel findings from motor behavior, temperament ratings and directional cardiac response. *Developmental Science,* 5, 441–51.

——. (2005). Behavioral approach-inhibition in toddlers: Prediction from infancy, positive and negative affective components, and relations with behavior problems. *Child Development,* 76, 212–26.

Vouloumanos, A., and Bryant, G. (2019). Five-month-old infants detect affiliation in co-laughter. *Scientific Reports,* 9 (1), 4158.

Sunscreen

AAD. (2018). Sunscreen FAQs. American Academy of Dermatology, https://www.aad.org/media/stats/prevention-and-care/sunscreen-faqs. Accessed August 2019.

AAP. (2019). Sun safety and protection tips. American Academy of Pediatrics, https://www.aap.org/en-us/about-the-aap/aap-press-room/news-features-and-safety-tips/Pages/Sun-Safety-and-Protection.aspx. Accessed August 2019.

Bray, F., et al. (2017). Sun protection for infants: Parent behaviors and beliefs in Miami, Florida. *Cutis,* 99, 339–41.

CDC. (2019). How can I protect my children from the sun? Centers for Disease Control and Prevention, https://www.cdc.gov/cancer/skin/basic_info/children.htm. Accessed August 2019.

Jemal, A., et al. (2005). Cancer statistics. *CA: A Cancer Journal for Clinicians,* http://CAonline.AmCancerSoc.org. Accessed August 2019.

Nazanin, F., et al. (2015). Sun protection for children: A review. *Journal of Pediatric Review,* 3 (1), e155.

Oliveria, S. A., et al. (2006). Sun exposure and risk of melanoma. *Archives of Disease in Childhood,* 91 (2), 131–38.

Paller, A. S., et al. (2011). New insights about infant and toddler skin: Implications for sun protection. *Pediatrics,* 128 (1), 92–102.

Saeedi, M. (2013). An overview of cosmetics and toiletries. Shelfin, Inc. In Nazanin, F., et al. (2015). Sun protection for children: A review. *Journal of Pediatric Review,* 3 (1), e155.

Strouse, J. J., et al. (2005). Pediatric melanoma: Risk factor and survival analysis of the Surveillance, Epidemiology and End Results Database. *Journal of Clinical Oncology,* 23, 4735–41.

Swaddling

CDC. (2018). Sudden unexpected infant death and sudden infant death syndrome. Centers for Disease Control and Prevention, https://www.cdc.gov/sids/about/index.htm. Accessed August 2019.

Harcke, H. T., et al. (2016). Sonographic assessment of hip swaddling techniques in infants with and without DDH. *Journal of Pediatric Orthopedics*, 36 (3), 232–38.

Horne, R. (2017). To swaddle or not to swaddle? International Society for the Study and Prevention of Perinatal and Infant Death, https://www.ispid.org/infantdeath/id-statements/swaddling. Accessed August 2019.

Loder, R. T., and Skopelja, E. N. (2011). The epidemiology and demographics of hip dysplasia. *International Scholarly Research Network Orthopedics*, 2011, 1–46.

Nelson, A. M. (2017). Risks and benefits of swaddling healthy infants: An integrative review. *MCN: The American Journal of Maternal/Child Nursing*, 42 (4), 216–25.

Pease, A. S., et al. (2016). Swaddling and the risk of sudden infant death syndrome: A meta-analysis. *Pediatrics*, 137 (6).

van Sleuwen, B. E., et al. (2007). Swaddling: A systematic review. *Pediatrics*, 120 (4), 1097–106.

Swimming

AAP. (2019). Swim lessons: When to start and what parents should know. American Academy of Pediatrics, https://www.healthychildren.org/English/safety-prevention/at-play/Pages/swim-lessons.aspx. Accessed August 2019.

Nguyen, B., and Warda, L. (2003). Swimming lessons for infants and toddlers. *Paediatrics and Child Health*, 8 (2), 113–19.

Sigmundsson, H., et al. (2010). Baby swimming: Exploring the effects of early intervention on subsequent motor abilities. *Child: Care Health and Development*, 36 (3), 428–30.

BIBLIOGRAPHY

Teaching Babies to "Read"

Courage, M. L., et al. (2016). Infants, toddlers and learning from screen media. *Encyclopedia on Early Childhood Development,* http://www.child-encyclopedia.com/technology-early-childhood-education/according-experts/infants-toddlers-and-learning-screen-media. Accessed August 2019.

Crespo, C. J., et al. (2001). Television watching, energy intake, and obesity in US children: Results from the third National Health and Nutrition Examination Survey, 1988–1994. *Archives of Pediatric and Adolescent Medicine,* 155 (3), 360–65.

DeLoache, J. S., et al. (2010). Do babies learn from baby media? *Psychological Science,* 21 (11), 1570–74.

Kearney, M. S., and Levine, P. B. (2015). Early childhood education by MOOC: Lessons from *Sesame Street*. NBER Working Paper no. 21229, National Bureau of Economic Research.

Linebarger, D. L., and Vaala, S. E. (2010). Screen media and language development in infants and toddlers: An ecological perspective. *Developmental Review,* 30 (2), 176–202.

Nathanson, A. I., et al. (2013). The relation between television exposure and theory of mind among preschoolers. *Journal of Communication,* 63 (6), 1088–1108.

———. (2014). The relation between television exposure and executive function among preschoolers. *Journal of Developmental Psychology,* 50 (5), 1497–1506.

Neuman, S. B., et al. (2014). Can babies learn to read? A randomized trial of baby media. *Journal of Educational Psychology,* 106 (3), 815–30. See this article for an exhaustive (and impressive) examination of the research available on the subject.

Teething Necklaces

AAP. (2018). Amber teething necklaces: A caution for parents. American Academy of Pediatrics, https://www.healthychildren.org/English/ages-stages/baby/teething-tooth-care/Pages/Amber-Teething-Necklaces.aspx. Accessed July 2019.

Abdulsatar, F., et al. (2019). Teething necklaces and bracelets pose significant danger to infants and toddlers. *Paediatrics and Child Health,* 24 (2), 132–33.

Cox, C., et al. (2017). Infant strangulation from an amber teething necklace. *Canadian Journal of Emergency Medicine,* 19 (5), 400–403.

CPS. (2015). Keep your baby safe: Caring for kids. Canadian Paediatric Society, http://www.caringforkids.cps.ca/handouts/keep_your_baby_safe. Accessed July 2019.

FDA. (2018). FDA warns about safety risks of teething necklaces, bracelets to relieve teething pain or to provide sensory stimulation. U.S. Food and Drug Administration, https://www.fda.gov/news-events/press-announcements/fda-warns-about-safety-risks-teething-necklaces-bracelets-relieve-teething-pain-or-provide-sensory. Accessed July 2019.

Soudek, L., and McLaughlin, R. (2018). Fad over fatality? The hazards of amber teething necklaces. *Paediatric Child Health,* 23 (2), 106–10.

Teething Numbing Gels

AAPD. (2012). Guideline on infant oral health care. *Pediatric Dentistry,* 34 (5), e148–52.

Chung, N. Y., et al. (2010). Severe methemoglobinemia linked to gel-type topical benzocaine use: A case report. *Journal of Emergency Medicine,* 38 (5), 601–6.

FDA. (2016). FDA recommends not using lidocaine to treat teething pain and requires new boxed warning. U.S. Food and Drug Administration, https://www.fda.gov/drugs/drug-safety-and-availability/fda-drug-safety-communication-fda-recommends-not-using-lidocaine-treat-teething-pain-and-requires. Accessed August 2019.

——. (2016). FDA warns against the use of homeopathic teething tablets and gels. U.S. Food and Drug Administration, https://www.fda.gov/news-events/press-announcements/fda-warns-against-use-homeopathic-teething-tablets-and-gels. Accessed August 2019.

——. (2018). Safely soothing teething pain and sensory needs in babies and older children. U.S. Food and Drug Administration, https://www.fda.gov/consumers/consumer-updates/safely-soothing-teething-pain-and-sensory-needs-babies-and-older-children. Accessed August 2019.

Lehr, J., et al. (2012). Benzocaine-induced methemoglobinemia in the pediatric population. *Pediatric Nursing,* 27 (5), 583–88.

Vohra, R., et al. (2017). Pediatric exposures to topical benzocaine preparations reported to a statewide poison control system. *Western Journal of Emergency Medicine,* 18 (5), 923–27.

Thumb Sucking

AAP. (2019). Thumbsucking. American Academy of Pediatrics, https://www.aap.org/en-us/about-the-aap/aap-press-room/aap-press-room-media-center/Pages/Thumbsucking.aspx. Accessed August 2019.

AAPD. (2019). Are thumb sucking and pacifier habits harmful for a child's teeth? American Academy of Pediatric Dentistry, https://www.aapd.org/resources/parent/faq/. Accessed August 2019.

Barbosa, C., and Fitzpatrick, A. L. (2009). The relationship of bottle feeding and other sucking behaviors with speech disorder in Patagonian preschoolers. *BMC Pediatrics,* 9, 66.

Borrie, F. R., et al. (2015). Interventions for the cessation of non-nutritive sucking habits in children. *Cochrane Database Systematic Reviews,* 16 (3), CD008694.

Ling, H., et al. (2018). The association between nutritive, non-nutritive sucking habits and primary dental occlusion. *BMC,* 18 (1), 145.

Mayo Clinic Staff. (2018). Thumb sucking: Help your child break the habit, https://www.mayoclinic.org/healthy-lifestyle/childrens-health/in-depth/thumb-sucking/art-20047038.aa2. Accessed August 2019.

Thumbsucking. (2019). Ask Dr. Sears, https://www.askdrsears.com/topics/parenting/discipline-behavior/bothersome-behaviors/thumbsucking. Accessed August 2019.

Tummy Time

AAP. (Last updated January 2017). Back to sleep, tummy to play. American Academy of Pediatrics, https://www.healthychildren.org/English/ages-stages/baby/sleep/Pages/Back-to-Sleep-Tummy-to-Play.aspx. Accessed August 2019.

——. (2019). Tummy time. American Academy of Pediatrics, https://www.aap.org/en-us/about-the-aap/aap-press-room/aap-press-room-media-center/Pages/Tummy-Time.aspx. Accessed August 2019.

Coleman, P. (2017). The strange reason tummy time was invented for babies. Fatherly, https://www.fatherly.com/health-science/tummy-time-reasons. Accessed August 2019. See this site for a clear and interesting narrative of the origins of tummy time.

Graham, J. (2006). Tummy time is important. *Clinical Pediatrics,* 45, 119–21.

Kadey, H. J., and Roane, H. S. (2012). Effects of access to a stimulating object on infant behavior during tummy time. *Journal of Applied Behavior Analysis,* 45 (2), 395–99. This article offers an excellent overview of the research available on the subject.

NIH. (Last updated 2013). Babies need tummy time! National Institutes of Health, https://safetosleep.nichd.nih.gov/safesleepbasics/tummytime. Accessed August 2019.

Vaccinations

AAP. (2018). Vaccine safety: The facts. American Academy of Pediatrics, https://www.healthychildren.org/English/safety-prevention/immunizations/Pages/Vaccine-Safety-The-Facts.aspx. Accessed August 2019.

CDC. (2012). If you choose not to vaccinate your child, understand the risks and responsibilities. Centers for Disease Control and Prevention, https://www.cdc.gov/vaccines/hcp/conversations/downloads/not-vacc-risks-color-office.pdf. Accessed August 2019.

——. (2017). Preventing and managing adverse reactions. Centers for Disease Control and Prevention, https://www.cdc.gov/vaccines/hcp/acip-recs/general-recs/adverse-reactions.html. Accessed August 2019.

——. (2019). Immunization schedules. Centers for Disease Control and Prevention, https://www.cdc.gov/vaccines/schedules/hcp/imz/child-adolescent.html?CDC_AA_refVal=https%3A%2F%2Fwww.cdc.gov%2Fvaccines%2Fschedules%2Feasy-to-read%2Fchild.html. Accessed August 2019.

Colorado Children's Immunization Coalition. (2019). Delayed schedule. http://www.immunizeforgood.com/fact-or-fiction/delayed-schedule. Accessed August 2019.

CPS. (2019). Immunization and vaccines. Canadian Paediatric Society, https://www.cps.ca/en/issues-questions/immunization. Accessed August 2019.

Doheny, K. (2014). Expert Q and A: Childhood vaccine safety. WebMD, https://www.webmd.com/children/vaccines/features/childhood-vaccine-safety#1. Accessed August 2019.

FDA. (2018). Thimerosal in vaccines questions and answers. U.S. Food and Drug Administration, https://www.fda.gov/vaccines-blood-biologics/vaccines/thimerosal-vaccines-questions-and-answers. Accessed August 2019.

Hambidge, S., et al. (2014). Timely versus delayed early childhood vaccination and seizures. *Pediatrics,* 133 (6), e1492–99.

Hviid, A., et al. (2019). Measles, mumps, rubella vaccination and autism: A nationwide cohort study. *Annals of Internal Medicine,* 170, 513–20.

Mayo Clinic Staff. (2013). Childhood vaccines: Tough questions, straight answers, https://www.mayoclinic.org/healthy-lifestyle/infant-and-toddler-health/in-depth/vaccines/art-20048334. Accessed August 2019.

NFID. (2019). Top reasons to get vaccinated. National Foundation for Infectious Diseases, http://www.nfid.org/about-vaccines/reasons. Accessed August 2019.

Oster, E. (2019). *Cribsheet*. New York. Penguin. See Oster's section on immunization-related risks for a clear and accessible explanation of the potential dangers.

Sears, R. W. (2007). *The Vaccine Book: Making the Right Decision for Your Child*. New York: Little, Brown.

Stratton, K., et al. (Eds.). (2011). *Adverse Effects of Vaccines: Evidence and Causality*. Washington, DC: National Academies Press.

United Nations Foundation. (2019). Vaccine-preventable diseases. Shot@Life, https://shotatlife.org/a-global-challenge/vaccine-preventable-diseases. Accessed August 2019.

U.S. Department of Health and Human Services. (2019). Vaccines.gov, https://www.vaccines.gov. Accessed August 2019.

WHO. (2012). If you choose not to vaccinate your child, understand the risks and responsibilities. World Health Organization, http://www.euro.who.int/_data/assets/pdf_file/0004/160753/If-you-choose_EN_WHO_WEB.pdf?ua=1. Accessed August 2019.

——. (2015). What are some of the myths—and facts—about vaccination? World Health Organization, http://www.euro.who.int/__data/assets/pdf_file/0005/339620/Myths-and-facts.pdf?ua=1. Accessed August 2019.

——. (2018). Immunizations, vaccines and biologicals. World Health Organization, https://www.who.int/immunization/documents/positionpapers/en. Accessed August 2019.

Vaping and Breastfeeding

AAP. (2019). Breastfeeding. American Academy of Pediatrics, https://www.aap.org/en-us/advocacy-and-policy/aap-health-initiatives/Breastfeeding/Pages/Benefits-of-Breastfeeding.aspx. Accessed August 2019.

Caldwell, A. L. (2019). E-cigarette use during pregnancy and breastfeeding FAQs. American Academy of Pediatrics, https://www.healthychildren.org/English/ages-stages/prenatal/Pages/E-Cigarette-Use-During-Pregnancy-Breastfeeding.aspx. Accessed August 2019.

CDC. (2018). Breastfeeding: Tobacco and e-cigarettes. Centers for Disease Control and Prevention, https://www.cdc.gov/breastfeeding/breastfeeding-special-circumstances/vaccinations-medications-drugs/tobacco-and-e-cigarettes.html. Accessed August 2019.

Chivers, E., et al. (2019). Nicotine and other potentially harmful compounds in "nicotine-free" e-cigarette liquids in Australia. *Medical Journal of Australia,* 210 (3), 127–28.

Czogala, J., et al. (2014). Secondhand exposure to vapors from electronic cigarettes. *Nicotine and Tobacco Research,* 16 (6), 655–62.

Flouris, A. D., et al. (2013). Acute impact of active and passive electronic cigarette smoking on serum cotinine and lung function. *Inhalation Toxicology,* 25 (2), 91–101.

Grana, R., et al. (2013). Background paper on e-cigarettes (electronic nicotine delivery systems). Center for Tobacco Control Research and Education, University of California, San Francisco, https://escholarship.org/uc/item/13p2b72n. Accessed August 2019.

Hayes, J. T. (2017). What is thirdhand smoke, and why is it a concern? Mayo Clinic, https://www.mayoclinic.org/healthy-lifestyle/adult-health/expert-answers/third-hand-smoke/faq-20057791. Accessed August 2019.

Matt, G. E., et al. (2011). Thirdhand tobacco smoke: Emerging evidence and arguments for a multidisciplinary research agenda. *Environmental Health Perspectives,* 119 (9), 1218–26.

Mennella, J. A., et al. (2007). Breastfeeding and smoking: Short-term effects on infant feeding and sleep. *Pediatrics,* 120 (3), 497–502.

Moore, B. F., et al. (2017). Exposure to secondhand smoke, exclusive breastfeeding and infant adiposity at age 5 months in the Healthy Start study. *Pediatric Obesity,* 12 (Suppl. 1), 111–19.

National Center for Chronic Disease Prevention and Health Promotion. (2016). 2016 Surgeon General's Report: E-cigarette use among youth and young adults. Centers for Disease Control and Prevention, https://www.cdc.gov/tobacco/data_statistics/sgr/e-cigarettes/index.htm. Accessed August 2019.

Walkers

AAP. (2001). Injuries associated with infant walkers. *Pediatrics,* 108 (3), 790–92.

Badihian, S., et al. (2017). The effect of baby walker on child development: A systematic review. *Iranian Journal of Child Neurology,* 11 (4), 1–6.

Sims, A., et al. (2018). Infant walker-related injuries in the United States. *Pediatrics,* 142 (4), https://pediatrics.aappublications.org/content/142/4/e20174332. Accessed August 2019.

Index

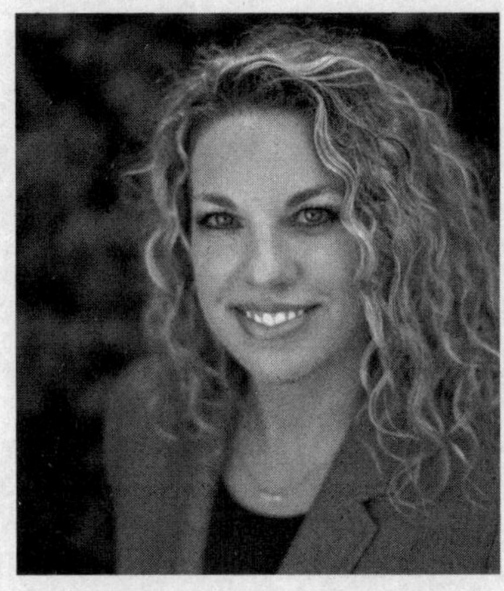

PHOTO: © DARRELL WALTERS

Tina Payne Bryson, Ph.D., is the founder and executive director of The Center for Connection, a multidisciplinary clinical practice in Southern California. She is the coauthor (with Daniel J. Siegel, M.D.) of two *New York Times* bestsellers, *The Whole-Brain Child* and *No-Drama Discipline,* as well as *The Yes Brain* and *The Power of Showing Up.* Dr. Bryson keynotes conferences and conducts workshops for parents, educators, and clinicians all over the world, and she frequently consults with schools, businesses, and other organizations. An LCSW, Tina is a graduate of Baylor University with a Ph.D. from USC. She lives in Los Angeles with her husband and three children.

TinaBryson.com
Facebook.com/TinaPayneBrysonPhD
Twitter: @tinabryson
Instagram: @tinapaynebryson

About the Type

The text of this book was set in Filosofia, a typeface designed in 1996 by Zuzana Licko, who created it for digital typesetting as an interpretation of the eighteenth-century typeface Bodoni, designed by Giambattista Bodoni (1740–1813). Filosofia, an example of Licko's unusual font designs, has classical proportions with a strong vertical feeling, softened by rounded droplike serifs. She has designed many typefaces and is the cofounder of *Emigre* magazine, where many of them first appeared. Born in Bratislava, Czechoslovakia, in 1961, Licko came to the United States in 1968. She studied graphic communications at the University of California, Berkeley, graduating in 1984.